A Primitive Diet

A book of recipes free from Wheat/Gluten, Dairy Products, Yeast and Sugar

For people with Candidiasis, Coeliac Disease, Irritable Bowel Syndrome, Ulcerative Colitis/ Crohn's Disease, Multiple Sclerosis, Asthma, Eczema, Psoriasis, Acne, Autism, food allergies and intolerances and those just wanting to become healthy

Beverley Southam

authorHOUSE®

AuthorHouse™ UK Ltd.
500 Avebury Boulevard
Central Milton Keynes, MK9 2BE
www.authorhouse.co.uk
Phone: 08001974150

Published by Beverley Southam -
in conjunction with AuthorHouse
'Pricklewood' Quinlans Road
QUAAMA NSW 2550
AUSTRALIA
Tel/Fax: 61 2 64938490
www.aprimitivediet.com.au

First published by AuthorHouse 8/18/2008

ISBN: 978-1-4343-4056-6 (sc)

Copyright Beverley Southam 2005, 2008.
Both books revised and combined as
A Primitive Diet in 2005
ISBN 0-9757 196-0-2
Printed in the United States of America
Bloomington, Indiana

This book is printed on acid-free paper.

A Primitive Diet First published 2001 Reprinted 2003
Cover design by Hippopotamus Dreams
SYDNEY AUSTRALIA.
Edited by : Motria Von Schreiber, Maggie Camfield, Geoffrey Southam

More of A Primitive Diet for Young and Old First published 2002

Disclaimer: Whilst the information contained in this publication has been formulated from
knowledge gained, personal experiences during my life and much personal research over
the past twenty five years, I have attempted to provide readers with basic information, and
urge them to take responsibility for their own health. For further help with their health
problems, I ask that they please seek the help of a qualified Naturopath or Herbalist.

"From food are born creatures,
which live upon food and after death return to food.
Food is the chief of all things. It is therefore said to be
the medicine of all diseases of the body."

The Upanishads c. 500 BC
(Vedic Literature - ancient sacred literature of the Hindus)

fresh raw foods, being alive, "give more strength".

Hippocrates 469 – 399 BC
Father of Medicine

"The Chinese do not draw any distinction
between food and medicine"

Lin Yut Ang

So…if our car operates on petrol, we don't fill
its tank with diesel do we, we know that it won't go.
Then why do we feed our body the wrong food and
assume it will keep going?

Beverley Southam.
Health + Happiness = Wealth

To All of You, I Say Thank You

Thank you to my husband, Geoffrey, for silently suffering my absences while I've been buried away in the shed typing, most times neglecting the dishes and laundry. I couldn't have done this without your love, encouragement and support. And I have to say, you make a great 'guinea pig' when it comes to trying out new recipes I dream up. But I promise, it's back to my domestic duties and the vegetable garden now!

Rebecca, our special daughter, what can I say...you started all this! Thank you for your input, the friendly disagreements we had over different health problems and nutrition, but it made us do more research and dig for more information to see who was right, didn't it? And, yes, I greatly respect you and admire you for the years of hard work to now hold a Bachelor of Health Science in Complementary Medicine. Please remember, the world desperately needs you and your knowledge.

Danny, our son, so tall and strong and gentle. Where are those doctors now, the doctors who told me you had Cystic Fibrosis or Coeliac Disease? It was my desperation seeing you so ill that led us down this path all those years ago. Here you are today, talented, a great sportsman, able to play music, sing and dance, the ability to do whatever you put your mind to, and a gentle leader. And I'm always so impressed to see you in the kitchen serving up a feast. Sorry too, Dan, that I passed on your Nanna's love of food!

Thank you, cousin Sue, your friendship is precious to me. At those times when I was doubting myself you seemed to pop up, hassling me for my recipes. The very encouragement I needed to keep on going.

Thank you so much Sandra Russett-Silk, for sharing your precious book on the Hunzas. It reassured me that we're walking the right path to eating and living a long healthy, happy and productive life. That trip to Hunza is still on when the time is right!

To Penny and Phil Wheater, much gratitude for your words of wisdom and the fantastic books you send us. Thank you Maggie and Motria for your valuable input.

Fay, your lesson in grinding and using fresh spices has induced me to add more to all sorts of dishes. Your recipes from the Middle East are delicious. I hope you don't mind but I had to include some in my book.

But most of all, this is in loving memory of my mother, Nona, who taught me from a very young age the fundamentals of a balanced, fresh food diet. I know you and Dad are with us everyday, smiling upon us, pleased that atleast one of your offspring learned from the lessons you tried to teach us.

So everyone, eat, be healthy and happy, and as Fay would say, "and enjoy".

Contents

FOREWORD

There is much recent debate about the impacts of agrichemicals on the environment and on human health. Over the last few years the excessive use of some pesticides had led to such speedy resistance in pest species that the manufacturers themselves are asking farmers to use smaller amounts. Run-off from such chemical use can enter water courses and may persist in soil and on the outside of fruit and vegetables for some considerable time. Livestock is also not immune. The extensive use of hormones, antibiotics and other treatments to prevent disease in over stocked conditions has led to concerns that these chemicals are entering the human food chain. Even fish are not exempt, with the stock in some fish farms effectively floating in a soup of nutrients and antibiotics. Changes have even been made to the milk available to most of us, with the rich creamy layered bottles of the past having been replaced with homogenised milk which has been suggested to contribute to circulatory disorders. In light of such changes to our food supply, it is little wonder that many people express concern about the possible impacts on human health.

Asthma, eczema, and an array of food allergies (especially wheat and dairy intolerance) all seem to be much more common today than in the recent past. Conditions such as irritable bowel disorder are also on the increase. Even our ability to reproduce may be under threat; concerns have been raised about the decrease in human sperm levels, with plasticisers, fungicides and pesticides being implicated. Obesity is becoming frequent in most urbanised societies.

Modern living conditions, including modern diets of highly processed foods containing high levels of sugar, salt and fats, are often implicated. However, medical opinion often seems divided about how to resolve these issues. Governments seem reluctant to challenge giant food and agrochemical industries, many of which have turnovers that are larger than some countries. Individuals can feel powerless. However, here is something that we can do as individuals to avoid some of these potential hazards: follow the advice in this book, go organic and eat a primitive diet. Luckily we do not need to suffer; the recipes that Beverley Southam has developed are not only healthy but tasty!

The logic of a primitive diet that replicates past experience seems sound: human evolution does not work fast enough to cope with major changes in food type over one or two generations. This book provides advice and a large number of good recipes based on foods that have featured in human diets for a considerable length of time. It is also encouraging that the author and her husband put their money where their instincts are and have swapped their comfortable suburban life for the excitement of developing a self-sufficient lifestyle based on growing their own produce in an organic and sustainable way.

We have enjoyed many of the recipes from this book, and felt the health benefits, and commend them to all who enjoy good healthy food.

Dr C. Philip Wheater
Principal Lecturer
Department of Environmental &
Geographical Sciences
Manchester Metropolitan University
Manchester UK

Dr Penny A. Cook
Senior Lecturer
Centre for Public Health
Liverpool John Moores University
Liverpool UK

INTRODUCTION

A Primitive Diet had its beginnings as leaflets of recipes for my daughter, Rebecca. The patients who came to her, at her naturopathic clinic, kept asking "but what can I eat?" So who else would you ring for help ... "Mum, send recipes, my patients need them!" I began typing. First they were going to be leaflets with recipes of foods I fed my family over the years, but one followed another, and I'd think, "Oh I'd better put this one in, and this one, and this one", and so it went on.

Many of Rebecca's patients suffered from allergies and food intolerances causing such illness, *Psoriasis*, gastrointestinal problems, *Asthma* and *Eczema*. While Rebecca advised them on nutrition, gave them herbs and watched with pleasure as they started to overcome their illnesses, they always had the problem of what to eat. There are lots of books out there on the market that are gluten-free, or yeast-free, or sugar-free or dairy-free, but it's so difficult to find any that leave out all these allergy-causing foods. And mostly the recipes are so bland and uninteresting, *and cooked!* Why do people think because they're on a special diet that it has to be boring? I know all this, because I was in the same position many years ago.

So, into the kitchen I would go and take things out of recipes, add things, change things around, make the dish then feed it to my family of wolves! They'd come into the kitchen and say, "Wow Mum, what's this? Oh, a Mummy thing," or "Oh, an ah la Southam". Friends began asking, "Is this a Bevvy thing?" Danny and Rebecca's friends were constantly coming and going at our house and I think it was always a bit of an adventure when it came to mealtimes.

Apart from the recipes, people continually ask why we eat so much raw food and live the way we do. I try not to bore them with details but for those who might be interested and will probably relate to our ordeal, I've included my family's story. With the dramatic escalation of diseases across the western world, I feel that perhaps I should impart a little of the knowledge gained over the years, by research, reading other people's experiences of overcoming disease, and my own experiences. Now, as well as diseases reaching epidemic proportions across the western world there is an added insult to Nature and Humanity with which to contend, the risk of Genetically Engineered/Modified foods.

"What qualifications do you have to be helping people with their diet?" I hear you ask. My only reply can be that the experience of life is often a better teacher than reading from a textbook or listening to a university lecture. People ask me for help to sort out their diet and their children's diet. One lady had problems with her two children who were hyperactive. We took away the chemicals, food preservatives, food colorings and they were put on a dairy-free, almost grain-free, fully balanced fresh raw fruit, vegetable, fish and nut diet. Within a week or two their nature changed so dramatically their mum couldn't believe the difference. One had suffered from bad croup for most of his nine years. The congestion broke up and was gone.

I've had lots of requests for recipes of bread replacements, treats to feed children and food for lunch boxes. I understand the big step to changing diet or in reality, a whole change of life style. Although any cooked food we personally eat is a special treat, or what I sometimes call a comfort food, I've included quite a number of these cooked food recipes for you to try. I've put suggestions for many of the recipes too, so that you get into the habit of adding and subtracting ingredients for variation, to get you going to making up your own recipes. BUT wean yourself off cooked food as soon as possible. A raw food diet is so simple, exciting and healthy.

I've added a small chapter about my study of the Hunzacuts, a group of people hidden away in a magnificent glacial valley in the Himalayan Mountains; and the life style and diet of the inhabitants of a group of islands in the South Pacific called the Marquesas. I was excited when I found that the diet on which we've lived for the last few years is along similar lines to these two old civilisations, and is more than adequate to nourish and sustain us long term.

Also I wanted to tell you about a few of the old simple remedies passed on by my grandparents and elderly neighbours who swore by them.

Some of them I still tend to use. *My wise grandmothers used fresh herbs and garlic in their food everyday and after giving it some thought, I believe they were unconsciously practising preventive medicine.*

Due to popular request I've included a shopping list to help stock the pantry and the refrigerator and I've added a section of healthy raw food that can be fed to babies. Once you adjust to thinking more raw fruits, vegetables, nuts and herbs, then the easier it will be to use your imagination and come up with delicious, healthy meals. After all these would have been the foods of Primitive Man.

I hope this brief outline of my life and that of my family assists you in some way, if you're bewildered by your lack of 'wellness'. I sincerely hope the diet and recipes help you on your way to optimum health.

A Primitive Diet

Okay, switch on your imagination please ... You've just stepped from a time machine. It's whizzed you back 6,000 years and you've stepped out into a lush green forest. Your survival will depend upon your ingenuity and commonsense.

Once you take in your surroundings, your stomach reminds you that you need food. What is there to eat? There's no McDonalds or café serving your favourite caffé latte in sight, but all around you there are real foods provided by Mother Nature, fresh, rich in nutrients, unpolluted, unprocessed, unmicrowaved (not cremated) and free from artificial fertilisers and chemicals. Juicy berries, fruits, nuts in their natural packaging are waiting to be cracked open, juicy greens abound. How easy is it? No cooking, no dishes to wash but more nutrition in one meal than you acquired from all your food of the previous week.

You eat your fill, you move on and look around. You hear water in the creek or running stream and decide you should have a drink. The water is delicious - unpolluted, free from chlorine, free from fluoride and full of minerals. There's a bird's nest with some eggs in. They're warm, should you eat them? Perhaps just one - it's best to leave some to hatch. You wander through this paradise in awe.

How simple our life could be if we returned to this way of eating - fresh, chemical-free, unprocessed, uncooked, organic food full of live nutrients and enzymes. The multibillion dollar *medical industry* would be out of work. The drug companies would have no human guinea pigs willing to test their latest dangerous experiments.

A Primitive Diet is the picture painted above. We eat very simple meals, predominantly raw, not quite as primitive man did but using the raw fruits, berries, vegetables, nuts, greens and herbs from his outdoor pantry. We eat eggs, often cooked, but also raw in dressings, smoothies, and as a dip for raw fish or raw sliced meat should we decide on a Japanese theme for dinner. We eat fish often, meat on a rare occasion for a special treat. My family has laughed at me for years because, when home alone for dinner I go to the vegetable garden and graze. I eat some leaves from the lettuces, a sprig of parsley, the heads from the broccoli, a carrot, a shallot, a radish, tomatoes if they are in season, then I go indoors and finish off with a handful of raw nuts, always with some form of fruit for dessert. If it's the right time of year I have strawberries, cape gooseberries or cossack pineapples (golden berries) in the garden. There I have a balanced meal. By eating the greens and nuts I have complete protein, plus calcium, magnesium and all the minerals through to the very necessary trace elements. The nuts give the all-important fats and oils my body requires. Carrots, broccoli and parsley, and the fruit give vitamin A/beta carotene, vitamin C and other essential vitamins and minerals, natural sugars, cellulose, roughage and of course the very purist form of water; live plants and fruits are more than 80% water. Afterward, I have no dishes to wash, dinner has cost me very little and my hunger is satisfied.

I know that you probably can't go to the garden and graze but you too can live a simple, healthy life as we do, beginning with a change in your diet and eating habits. Always strive to buy certified organic fruits and vegetables. This will help you avoid the genetically engineered/ modified foods, chemical sprays, artificial fertilizers, irradiation and lack of nutrients in normal supermarket produce. The argument that people can't afford to buy them is very shallow when you stand at supermarket checkouts and watch the food packets from the shopping trolleys as they pass through the register - frozen pizzas, frozen dinners, cakes, pies, chocolates, the ever present bottle of coca cola or cordial. I always buy organic and my shopping bill is less than half that of these people; half the food bill, it eliminates the medical bills, and enriches our lives. I see people spend as much or more on a block of chocolate and a packet of biscuits than I spend buying enough apples to last two of us for the week. A couple I helped with a diet change had a drop in their food bill from more than $200 a week to $150 and her husband has already been able to throw away the drugs he was taking. His supposed medical condition had mysteriously disappeared. Incidentally our weekly food bill rarely goes over $150, and we eat large meals with snacks of dried fruits and nuts in between.

You will notice that through my description of a primitive diet I haven't mentioned grains. We eat almost no grain except as a treat or a 'comfort' food. Humans are not meant to eat grain and have only been attempting to make them edible for human consumption since we became agriculturalists 4,000 - 6,000 years ago. This is not enough time for our digestive system to have adapted to digest grain.

There are those who argue with us about our raw, ***primitive diet***. They feel they have the knowledge, or university qualifications and our diet contradicts what the doctors, nutritionists and dietitians say. Who wrote these courses and texts from which they learn at university? How old are the texts? On what research have they based their advice and information? More important, who paid for the research? Was any of the research based on personal experience?

Dr Norman Walker was busy curing people of diseases as long ago as the late 1930s and 40s after first curing himself of acute neuritis by eating raw fruits, vegetables, their juices and nuts. It was the ordinary people, just like us today, who took notice and began climbing their way back to health. From the moment I picked up my little book written by Dr Walker, explaining the difference between live food and dead food, our lives changed forever. His book on raw foods made such simple commonsense. Through his research he proved conclusively that raw food was the correct food to nourish our body. With cooking, once our fruit and vegetables reach a temperature of 130°F our food is dead, its live elements and enzymes are destroyed or rendered difficult for our body to digest. Makes sense doesn't it? Then consider this, do we see cows, sheep or goats cooking their food? Where do they find their nutrition? In fresh, raw grass. What about bears, tigers, kangaroos, koalas or our first cousins, the gorillas? Who cooks their meals? Our very large cousins, the gorillas eat a straight vegetarian, grain-free diet, so why don't we? Perhaps our cousins have a superior knowledge and wisdom to us.

Max Gerson of Germany was another advocate of a raw food diet early last century. He used diet and raw vegetable juices to cure people of disease in Europe. One such person was Dr Albert Schweitzer who he cured of severe diabetes.

Not long after embarking on our new raw food diet I happened upon some more information that proved to me conclusively that we were on the right path. Have you ever heard of Pottenger's Cats? In the 1930s and 1940s, Dr Francis Pottenger was conducting operations on cats and trialing biological extracts. He was puzzled at the mortality rate amongst his laboratory cats. He believed he fed them well so that they would be in optimum health for his experiments. He fed them cooked meat scraps of liver, heart, brains (the offal), raw milk and cod liver oil. He was confused by the poor condition of his cats, which made them poor subjects for his research. He found that his cats were showing deficiencies, and each generation of kittens was being born with more and more deformities. As more cats were handed to him, he needed to find another supplier for more meat scraps. This supplier's meat scraps were raw. He fed these scraps to the second group of cats he took in, so one group was fed cooked meat, the second group fed raw. The second group of cats began to show improved health. This accidental discovery called for further experimentation.

Dr Pottenger studied 900 cats over a period of ten years coming up with some very conclusive results. He found that the cats fed cooked food began to deteriorate in health. They suffered through difficult labours and often had no milk for their kittens who were beginning to show deformities. Some cats never became pregnant. Miscarriages increased. The female cats grew more irritable and vicious while the toms became lazy, docile and lacking in sexual aggression. They all developed allergies, infections, sores, ulcers and tumors, and were plagued by fleas and internal parasites. *__Has the human race now slipped this low too?__*

The cats fed raw food produced healthy kittens from generation to generation, and showed none of the problems of those who ate cooked food. They were strong and free of all the health problems, and mothers contentedly fed their kittens as Nature intended.

Dr Pottenger furthered his experiments with the degenerating kittens. He took a number of them and began feeding them raw food. Their health improved dramatically but it took up to four generations to return the cats to excellent health.

Pottenger with his experiments on his 900 cats was criticised, and his results were not taken seriously by the scientific community. It was argued that cats were not human beings, but we are both mammals are we not? And we are all animals are we not? Animals totally out of step with Mother Nature and our world around us. The results of Dr Pottenger's cat experiments and their possible relevance to human nutrition should have been further investigated, but his work was merely swept aside.

So now you will understand why I am suggesting we eat raw food, as our primitive ancestors did. Any time you have a question about food or medicine, ask yourself, "What would Primitive Man have done?"
I realise there are a number of cooked food recipes in this book, and you will now understand why we class these as 'comfort foods'. For us they are foods we have as a special treat, or when friends come for a meal. They don't form part of our everyday diet. I've included the gluten-free rice/corn pasta, rice noodles, breads and dampers, cakes and biscuits due to popular request, and because we know how difficult it is to change old habits. As you eat more raw food you will see your health improve, and that will give you the confidence to become more adventurous in your eating.

I've seen some impressive results with two different people in the last few weeks. A fellow with whom we've just become acquainted, was being pressured by doctors into having his bowel removed due to severe intestinal problems. After four weeks on a total change of diet he saw his health improve beyond all his expectations. He still has a long way to go but he doesn't require further proof that he is on the right path. A desperate young mother has seen the turn around of her small son, who in my opinion was showing signs of autism. He had lost his ability to speak, his powers of communication, and had developed behavioural problems. His diet was changed to eating avocadoes, lots of carrots and carrot juice, fruits, greens and any raw food his mum could convince him to eat. Within six to eight weeks he began to talk clearly and communicate again, his behavior changed and he has now taken his place back in his family.

Are you convinced? So what are you waiting for, why not try it for yourself?

Our Story

Where does one begin, or better still how does one begin?

I began life in Narooma, a small seaside town on the far south coast of NSW, Australia, sleeping my babyhood away in the cane clothes basket. I was number four of six children. My fourth birthday I celebrated in an isolation ward in Camperdown Children's Hospital, Sydney, fighting meningitis. I recovered and was able to return home to the bush where not long afterwards I contracted a bad case of measles, but once over this setback I had the immune system of an ox. I was one of those fit, skinny kids that ran around summer and winter with no shoes and almost no clothes on. My mum called me 'Skinny Minnie' and was forever telling me to put on a jacket. I rarely caught colds and suffered no other childhood illnesses.

At 15 I discovered milkshakes. My girlfriends and I would walk downtown to Sam's Café. Sam made the best malted milkshakes in town. We'd sit in a booth drinking and listening to the juke box while watching the local 'talent' coming in and out. It was about this time that I developed chronic hayfever, sinus and a hint of asthma and began to have sick days from school. I managed to pass my Year 10 School Certificate exams without effort and as there was no chance for me to continue on with Years 11 and 12, I left and went to work. At 17 I found I had a weeping breast and because I was incredibly shy, especially about my body, I was too embarrassed to talk to anyone, so I had no idea that there could be a more serious problem. Finally, after about four months I told Mum about it while getting tea ready one night. Poor Mum. She sent me straight to the doctor. Within a week or two I was operated on and had a breast tumor removed, which I assume to this day was benign since I didn't bother to find out the results. No doubt the doctors would have informed me if it had been malignant, but basically I'd never heard of breast cancer. I had only become aware of cancer because I'd overheard Mum and Dad talk of a man in town who'd died from it.

At 19 I married my husband, Geoff, my buddy and support for the past

32 years. Geoff had been a bit of a rolling stone when I met him but he decided it was time to settle into a permanent job, learning to make cheese at the little ABC Cheese Factory at Central Tilba. So began our adventures into the world of cheese. I'd eaten very little cheese before that so it was a new taste sensation.

Three years later the first baby was on the way. I was 22. The plan was that we would have children while we were young so we could play with them and grow with them, then they'd be off out into the world while we would be in our 40's and still young enough to enjoy ourselves. We were so excited but appendicitis flared. The doctor wouldn't believe that it was serious, his religious beliefs overrode any judgement of my condition, and he believed he had to save the baby at all costs. Unfortunately one night it was too much so Geoff drove me 40 minutes to hospital where I was admitted. The following day my doctor and his colleague had an argument over my condition. I couldn't eat without being ill, the pain hadn't gone away but my doctor felt I was acting. On Tuesday, the surgeon who visited once a month was brought into the fray and he decided there and then to remove my appendix. First we had a chat during which he told me that if I lost my baby it was because Mother Nature was taking care, that it had possibly been poisoned by my appendix. Three nights later I miscarried.

Not to be put off, we started again and along came an 3.71kg / 8lb3oz baby Rebecca who entered the world exhausted after 36 hours in a labour ended by caesarean birth. Of course I was treated heavily with antibiotics on the chance I may develop an infection. Breastfed Rebecca received a good dose as well, passed on in my milk so I took home a very colicky baby. (Thanks to Dr Patrick Kingsley and his book *Foods That Conquer Cystitis* we now know that colic is caused by *Candida* yeast overgrowth). We battled the colic with Rebecca for three months, until it disappeared and we settled into a more regular routine.

As life went on, due to both a love of cooking taught to me by my mum and my new discovery of milk and cheese, I cooked with milk and cheese, I experimented with milk and cheese and I have to admit I was hooked. Healthwise my hayfever and sinus were worse and I was having severe bouts of tonsillitis. When Rebecca was eight months old it was decided that I should have my tonsils removed before trying for another baby so I was booked in for the surgeon's next monthly visit. All went well, my tonsils were removed and I just had to recover. I went home to the farm five days after the operation but then while sitting at the dinner table eating a very soft poached egg, I began to haemorrhage from the throat. Geoff in a state of panic rang for the ambulance and I was on a speedy trip back to the hospital. On arrival, two of the doctors made a decision to take me to theatre and somehow mend my throat, so I was anaesthetised in preparation but when I awoke I found myself back in the ward, they'd done nothing because neither was a qualified surgeon. My doctor then put me on morphine. I was told it was to help the blood clot so for five more days I lay, having horrific hallucinations, drifting in and out of consciousness. Only Geoff was allowed to visit me. On the fifth day my bladder muscles collapsed and the nursing sisters called in the doctor on duty. He used a catheter to relieve me, morphine was stopped and slowly I made it back onto my feet three days before Christmas.

Three months later I miscarried another baby. I coped better this time because I held the belief that if I lost a baby then it was possible there was something wrong, and Nature was taking care of it. Three days on I left hospital. I felt I had to escape. Geoff and I had planned a holiday and I had never been on a holiday like this before, we were going to Queensland.

Still not fully recovered, while staying at Yepoon I came down with a massive attack of *cystitis*. I'd never had an attack so bad before. They continued to plague me for the next few years until I discovered it was largely due to *Candida* yeast overgrowth and food intolerances made worse by large doses of antibiotics.

Three months further along Danny was on the way and we were really excited once more. All went well. I was always a very fit pregnant lady, I never suffered morning sickness or other problems that can develop during pregnancy. I think my youth and fitness (I frequently walked the paddocks with my mother-in-law, helping to check on the cows) and my healthy attitude contributed to this fitness. The gynaecologist thought this baby was going to be small but still it should be born by caesarean so 3.6kgs / 8lb1½ oz Danny came into the world. I was dosed with antibiotics again 'just in case'. Breastfeeding Danny at this moment was a very unwise decision, but it's easy to see things in hindsight, although if I had been wiser I would have refused the antibiotics. So I fed him one end and it passed right out the other, the antibiotics were going straight through him. Next major error, Danny had to be put on formula before I left the hospital so I took home another extremely colicky baby with a snuffliness and a rattle when he breathed. The doctor told me he could have breathed in some mucous when he was born, but it would soon go. It turned into severe bronchial asthma and nights were spent holding him upside down in the bathroom, the hot tap in the shower running to create steam to try to clear his airways. Later we came up with the scathingly brilliant idea of boiling the electric frypan beside his bed to make steam. He was continually with ear, nose and throat infections and rashes or dry patches of skin. He was having dose after dose of antibiotics. At ten months of age the family doctor said he wanted to refer Danny to a paediatrician at Canberra hospital. He believed him to have *Cystic Fibrosis* or *Coeliac Disease* because of his 'failure to thrive'. I honestly didn't believe this was the case but went to prove them wrong. For a week they did many nasty tests including threading a tube down Danny's throat to his stomach with a tiny camera attached. By the end of the week I drove home with a terrified, clinging baby and the knowledge that "we're very sorry Mrs Southam, we couldn't find anything wrong". So life went on.

In the meantime I took myself to the hospital and had small tumors cut from the end of my knitting finger. Life was never dull. Through all this we were trying to live a 'normal' life, going fishing, surfing and having picnics, all the family things, on Geoff's one day off from work each week.

My 57 year old mother, our support team of one, died of a cerebral haemorrhage two weeks before Danny turned one year old. We were told that the side effects of her high blood pressure medication her doctor had prescribed for her for a number of years, had weakened the arterial walls. As her pressure was elevated, the artery to her brain burst. It left our little family devastated but it's incredible what strength one can find when it's needed.

One Sunday night at fourteen months of age, Danny went into violent convulsions and was rushed off to hospital for four days. During his stay I had an angry confrontation in the hospital corridor with the doctor who virtually accused me of being a bad mother, I should have known Danny had an inner ear infection. Following this it was discussed with us about inserting drains or grommets in his ears. Then a week later Rebecca developed tonsillitis. They had given her some trouble on and off so she was booked in to have her adenoids and tonsils removed. By now I was stretched to the limit and I had taken to sleeping in an old beanbag beside Rebecca's bed at night, waiting for her fever to break. I was fearful of her also going into convulsions.

Before Geoff set out for work one morning I decided that I needed the car to get out of home for the day and have a break in routine. I dressed the three of us and drove an hour south to Bega, the nearest large town, where we drifted in and out of shops. I had no money to spend, we were extremely poor. We'd moved to a small holiday cottage on the outskirts of Narooma, and sometimes we only had $20 left for the week to buy food. We were surviving on our home grown vegetables and fruit, fish and of course milk and cheese.

In Bega as I my wandered along the line of shops I noticed a sign pointing to an office, it had 'Naturopath' on it. I'd seen a segment of *The Mike Walsh Show* on TV once where he interviewed a naturopath and a mum with her son. The naturopath hadn't claimed to cure the boy but by prescribing certain herbs, vitamins and minerals and lots of raw vegetable juices, he'd built up the boy's immune system to overcome a malignant bone tumor on his thighbone. After all kinds of therapy he'd been given just weeks to live and that's where the naturopath took over. The boy made a complete recovery. With all of this running through my mind, and before I had time to change it, I went into the waiting room and asked to see the naturopath. I was given an appointment for two that afternoon so for the next couple of hours I walked the shops asking myself, "Should I or shouldn't I?" During the 70's and 80's naturopaths were still regarded as 'Quacks' but two o'clock found me in with the naturopath. She used Iridology to read their eyes, she asked many questions and at the end of it all she told me that "basically you have two healthy kids, but you have to take them off dairy foods". I remember my reaction vividly. I was stunned. What was I going to feed them? She told me fruits, vegetables, eggs, fish, but not dairy food. She handed me bottles of herbal medicines to give them and said that in about three to four days, Danny in particular would develop a running nose, a cough and probably even mucous in his nappy as the herbs cleaned out his clogged up system. I drove home with all this new information going round and round in my head.

That night I sat the herbal medicines in front of Geoff saying, "Guess what I did today" and started explaining. Being dubious, he brought out the dictionary and looked up the list of ingredients written on the bottles. At the end we'd found that they contained herbs, vitamins and minerals, and as far as we could see nothing that would be detrimental to the kids.

On cue, four days later Danny's nose began to run with thick mucous and he developed a cough. My initial reaction was "Now what?!" then I remembered the naturopath's warning. Poor Danny, I followed him around mopping at his nose till it was red and sore. I caught him wiping it up the sleeve of his jumper and he coughed and croaked. Ten days later, while we watched TV we realised we couldn't hear Danny breathing as he slept. He'd always had a loud, raspy breathing. We both rushed into the bedroom and stood over him. He lay totally at peace, sleeping as he had never slept before, no rasping, no snoring nor croaking. It brought tears of relief to both of us.

Another comment that comes to mind - the naturopath suggested that Danny was a poor eater and I had to admit that yes he was. She told me that once his system was cleaned out of all the mucous clogging it up, he'd begin to eat and eat anything we put on his plate. Never was a truer word spoken. From that time Danny and Rebecca always ate large meals and anything served up, even their fresh vegetable juices they drank without question because they knew that this was their medicine.

Rebecca picked up fast as well, and when it was time for her tonsil operation we proudly declared that she no longer required it. Just one small disappointment though, the antibiotics she had been given for her tonsillitis had decayed two of her baby teeth. Thank heaven later they were replaced with her adult teeth.

A bit of a misunderstanding that occurred a year or two down the track proved to us everything we had learned that year. Danny, at preschool one morning was accidentally given a cup of milk for little lunch. By nightfall he had developed a severe asthma attack. We'd had no need to visit the naturopath once the kids were well again, and she had actually moved away. Because we had no one to go to in an emergency we went to our family doctor. He prescribed a bottle of red bronchial mixture which made Danny sleep but did nothing to improve his condition. In disgust I threw it out and mixed up a cup of honey, lemon juice and glycerine. Each time I thought he needed it I gave him a spoonful. Within hours his wheezing started to loosen and in a couple of days he was well on the way to being normal again. Next visit to the doctor I chided him for giving me the medicine. He asked what I'd done so I told him about the honey, lemon and glycerine. His comment was "Good for you. Don't you know that cough mixture is 95% glycerine anyway?"

While things were running smoothly for the rest of the family I miscarried another baby and found myself back in hospital for a curettage. I was woken from the anaesthetic by the doctor taking my blood pressure and my pulse which he did every half hour. The following morning I could barely move. I felt as though I was bruised all over, so I questioned the doctors on their rounds. They informed me that I'd had a cardiac arrest on the operating table and they'd had trouble bringing me round. They couldn't find a reason for this except perhaps I'd had a reaction to the anaesthetic. I think by this time my body was tired of living. We decided then that two babies would bring us as much joy as four so there was to be no more.

Life flowed so smoothly from there on. Because I had to change Rebecca and Danny's diet, I found it much easier to change ours also. By eliminating dairy foods, mysteriously my hayfever and sinus disappeared and I began to feel better. Around this time the dairy company that Geoff worked for, in their wisdom sold off the little cheese factory at Central Tilba and Geoff who had been manager there for seven years, was transferred to Bega.

Stresses of moving away from everything with which I was familiar, I suppose you could say stepping out of my comfort zone, once again played havoc with my health. I knew no one in Bega and because I was painfully shy I was not very good at going out and making friends. Arthritis, the legacy of my near crippled grandmother started in my ankle and wrist. My stomach started to bloat and I developed pain in my side. I looked up a recommended doctor and paid him a visit. He told me to take aspirin for the arthritis and when it was too bad come back for stronger medication. The pains in my side he suggested weren't really serious. He felt that when he pressed into my stomach I should have "nearly jumped off the couch". I decided to put up and shut up but that was a bit difficult, sometimes, the pain was quite severe. Then I discovered a lump once again in my left breast and I called on the next recommended doctor on my list. I was very impressed with his response. Rather than cut the lump out he suggested that I should visit the breast clinic in Sydney. A biopsy and mammogram were taken and the whole experience restored my faith in the medical profession. I was treated with such respect and kindness and they were able to give me some results then and there. I was advised that the tumor was benign, but to keep a check to see that it didn't change size or shape. It's still there after 22 years but I have no concern for it. I feel confident that with my nil intake of dairy foods and especially red meat, and with our high consumption of raw food, carrot and other raw vegetable juices, I'm not under any threat.

The next major dietary change came after doing the weekly shopping one morning. I'd stopped by a bookstand in the local supermarket and glanced down the books. The title *Raw Vegetable Juices - What's Missing in Your Body* by Dr Norman W.Walker D.Sc. immediately caught my attention. On flicking through, some of the words and chapter titles jumped off the pages at me, all sounding full of commonsense. The book went straight into my shopping trolley. It cost me just $2.00.

That small paperback became like a bible to me. It explained that our bodies are made of billions of microscopic cells all needing live nourishment so we should feed them live food, once food reaches 130*F it is no longer alive. I read about raw carrots and their incredible properties, spinach/silverbeet, cabbage, an excellent cleanser of the stomach and intestinal tract, garlic one of our most valuable food medicines of all. The more I read the more it sounded good, simple commonsense. When I read the chapter "Oh! So You Have a Cold Have You?" blaming dairy food as partly being responsible for the common cold, it all re-enforced what the naturopath had said.

My weekly shopping day became a new adventure, buying raw nuts, baskets full of fresh fruit and a few top-up vegetables that we didn't have in the garden at the time. The weight I had gained while being pregnant with Danny virtually 'fell off' and I went back to being my normal self. The kids were excellent, they always ate what was in front of them and right from an early age they ate as much as Geoff and I. I did get annoyed a number of times when they visited their friends' homes because the mums would dish out foods like ice cream and when our kids politely declined they'd be told "But this little bit won't hurt". I always knew if they'd had some, they'd get a bit of a cough and Danny would get a touch of eczema around the mouth or ear. Out would come the lemon, honey and glycerine mixture to the rescue.

Both of our children had enormous powers of concentration and excelled at school. They were always so calm and had excellent memories. They both loved sport and the outdoors which we always tried to share with them. By the age of 14 Danny had a state and Australian ranking as a junior tennis player. To tournaments we would take bags of fruit, especially bananas which are full of potassium, and we made him glasses of raw vegetable juices to sustain him. We watched while other players ate hamburgers, big Macs, chocolate bars and drank coke and thick shakes. Their concentration would lapse and their power would be gone while Danny just ploughed on. Cricket was his other passion. Rebecca played tennis, hockey, netball and even had a go at water polo, but she especially excelled at dancing, music and singing. They never came down with any of the 'bugs' that went around, we never had sleepless nights or interrupted sleep. Life with our young people was our greatest joy, we laughed and cried and shared everything as a family. Our life was special, we were pretty poor but money couldn't buy what we had. The only regret I have is that my mum couldn't be around to see them grow up, though I feel she's there giving a silent helping hand all the way.

In November 1985 I was offered a part time job. By now the kids were 7 and 9 and we felt it was okay for me to start back in the workforce. Over the years to help out with the finances I decorated wedding cakes, 21st birthday cakes and the likes and baby-sat children while their mothers were at work. In the early days in Narooma I wrote and had printed a cheese recipe book of all things, of which we sold a few thousand. Now was the time for me to go back to work.

After fifteen months I was moved to full time and with the stresses of the job back came my most dreaded enemy, *Cystitis*. I'd just finish one round of antibiotics and it would be back so I'd be on another. Following the fourth bout the doctor referred me to the gynaecologist while saying he wanted to put me on antibiotics for six months. The gynaecologist could find nothing wrong gynaecologically but both doctors had a large disagreement over me, so I had to find another doctor. I had kidney x-rays, cystoscopies, colonoscopies, laparoscopies. I went through seven doctors and three surgeons. The reports all told me that I was physically fit! Then what was wrong? I was now only 7stone 9lb in weight and I knew I was sick. I visited a female doctor while having an attack of *Cystitis*, hoping she would be sympathetic and give me a couple of days off to get over it but she told me that it was a female problem, some women develop it, and I was stuck with it.

The last doctor I visited was the registrar of King George V Hospital for Women in Sydney. He spent the best part of two hours of his own time on a Saturday morning seeing me. He was also baffled and wanted to perform a laparoscopy. I went back to Sydney for it the next week. He told me all was fine, but he was puzzled. I'd had *Endometriosis* at some time but it had gone leaving scars as evidence. We knew it had to be the vegetable juices and our diet especially without dairy food, a known causative factor in *Endometriosis*. A previous surgeon told me I had a problem that only elderly men get, a narrowing of the opening from the bladder and every year or two I would need to go into hospital to have it stretched. He'd actually done that while he was performing a cystoscopy on me and he had torn me about. The pain of passing urine for the next few days was excruciating. My doctor from King George V Hospital decided, though not qualified, he would undertake his own cystoscopy after he performed the laparoscopy and he told me it was bunkum, there was nothing wrong with my bladder. I was becoming desperate. As Geoff and I sat in front of TV one evening I said to him quietly how peaceful it would be to be dead. He looked so scared but I assured him I was too much of a coward and had no wish to do myself any harm.

Then the enormous itchy welts began spreading over my body, when they joined up I would collapse and have to lie about for atleast three days till the attack passed. My feet and hands or my face would swell, my temperature would soar and often the cramps in my stomach doubled me over with acute pain as though with a bowel blockage. One particular morning I remember well, I was in such a mess, my feet were swollen so I couldn't walk and I was doubled with severe stomach cramps. Geoff drove me to the casualty ward at the hospital and carried me in. The sister on duty looked at us both and said, "Sorry luv, you're better off going to yer own doctor later", so Geoff carried me back to the car and we drove home. I eventually managed to see the doctor in his surgery and he told me it was just an attack of *gastroenteritis* but before I left he made me take Panadol for the raging temperature. In the 15 minutes it took to reach home the Panadol had caused a hot prickly rash all over my body. The episodes of welts and cramps came often. Twice I collapsed on Rebecca while Geoff was away travelling to tennis tournaments with Danny. The first time I fell backward into the bath while taking a shower but fortunately I had the presence of mind to turn off the shower before I went down. At times like these the kids would help make the meals and feed them to me while I lay on the lounge. They helped with the washing, the ironing and the vacuuming.

It was a friend I worked with who finally discovered what was wrong with me. One morning she rushed in through the office very excited, waving a small newspaper clipping and calling out " I think I know what's wrong with you!" That's when I first became aware of *Candida albicans*, to be correct, *Candidiasis*.

Candida albicans is a yeast mould found living normally on the skin and in the mucous membranes of humans. While the body is healthy it's under control but once the balance is upset and our defences are down it invades. Doctors recognise it only as thrush, a condition of the female genital tract or the white curd-like deposit in a baby's mouth that cannot be wiped away. Because _Candida_ has so many symptoms doctors have little understanding of it. They're taught to prescribe to symptoms, rarely how to get to the bottom of a problem. In actual fact _Candida_ can affect every organ of the body. Our health, or defences (immune system), is continually under attack by what we eat, processed foods, chemicals around us, in our food and polluting our environment, drugs and antibiotics, both prescribed for us and injected or fed to animals we eat.

My research began. I read every book I could find. I found another naturopath in Canberra to help me. She had a pathologist take a blood sample, place it under a microscope with a monitor then explained everything she found in my blood. She pointed out the black *Candida* in my blood. It was then that I discovered how important our liver is to us. I was first and foremost given a liver tonic to pick me up, and went on an elimination diet cutting out foods like dairy (I was still sneaking cream onto my food). I removed wheat flour, the second most allergy causing food and other glutinous grains. Miraculously the welts disappeared, slowly my bowel functioned normally again and I was feeling exceptionally good. Thanks to our daughter, Rebecca, I found a book thrown on a bargain table in a local bookshop that explained everything clearly. The book was *Foods That Conquer Cystitis - The effective new way to treat Cystitis, Candida and Thrush* by Dr Patrick Kingsley, a very experienced clinical ecologist, written with the support of his colleagues in Canada and Great Britain. I studied it closely. It explained things I already knew and much more but until now I didn't understand. That's when I realised more of the benefits of *A Primitive Diet* and knew this was the way Nature intended for us to live. Dr Kingsley's book became my second bible.

And here I am today, the fittest and healthiest I've been since my teens. I'm acutely aware of the food I put into my mouth, of chemicals and our surrounding environment. In Bega our whole suburban garden was organic and free of any harmful chemicals. We saw the return of the good bugs to control the bad bugs and we had butterflies back in our garden. We grew our fruits and vegetables and dried our fruits for the winter. We bought as little as possible unless we could buy organic foods or know from where our food came. We also grew our herbs for our medicine and teas. We hope the day will come when doctors go back to treating people naturally with proper diet and herbs, and stop being controlled by the World's powerful drug companies. Rebecca once said while nursing me through one of my 'bouts' on the lounge, "Mum, one day I'm going to make you well and you'll never be sick ever, ever again." Today she is out in the community as a naturopath with first hand knowledge and an enormous awareness of how foods and our environment have such an impact on our wellbeing. Our son, Danny has even been heard to advise a friend to give up her dairy food and her bronchitis would go away. These days he's tall and well built at 1.9mtrs / 6ft3ins with bones like steel and teeth … he has never had a reason to visit the dentist. He grew up without dairy foods and little meat, eating mostly fish, raw nuts and eggs, not forgetting fresh raw fruits and vegetables.

Our latest threat we're now tackling is Genetically Modified/ Engineered foods. They are being rushed into our food chain and

it's an enormous possibility they'll be the cause of mass destruction of our human race. Why experiment with mice and rats if the biotechnologists can experiment on humans!

Over three years ago Geoff and I made another tough decision and the next phase of our life has begun. We sold our suburban home of 20 years where we raised our children and we've risked all. We've bought land to grow organic/biodynamic fruits, vegetables, nuts and medicinal herbs, including some native produce, to be sold in the local market place. The world of tomorrow is going to need all the help it can get. We believe that it's going to have to revert to the local market gardener or farmer to supply fresh, organic produce to the local market not the almighty, powerful supermarkets. This is already happening in many countries across Europe, and USA. Great Britain is so fortunate that they have Prince Charles and his estate as an excellent example and inspiration, to show the way farming should be done. His whole estate is farmed organically. Conventional agriculture will have to return to traditional farming if we are to survive the world of tomorrow.

So here we are in our new life, living in our little one room cabin with its bush shower and toilet just making ends meet, but as a team we'll do it. It's very rewarding and peaceful working the land to the rhythm of the moon, the planets and Nature. And we're happy in the knowledge that we're making our small contribution to the world of tomorrow, to hopefully leave something behind for our children and grandchildren.

What...No Dairy Foods?!!!

Question 1. **What animal on this planet other than humans, consume the milk and its manufactured products, of another animal, especially after having been weaned from one's own mother's milk?** No other creature.

Question 2. **What do grown up cows, goats and sheep eat?** Their nourishment comes from live plants, not milk and their processed by-products, nor cooked foods.

Thinking back to life in the bush, as a child with a mum who was an excellent cook, it was never impressed on us that we had to drink milk or eat any other milk-related products. Mum's emphasis was on eating fruit and vegies.

Each morning we were up by 7 o'clock. We were dressed, our beds made, and all of us were at the table for a full breakfast of cereal with a dash of milk, (I never was fond of the stuff), eggs or tomatoes on toast. If we weren't the 'right age' to drink a cup of tea, we would mostly finish with a drink of water. Snacks were fruit, or on a rare occasion we would be allowed a biscuit. Lunch was really dinner. We had our cooked meal of freshly picked vegetables and fruit at 12.30 when Dad came home for lunch and we came from school. Tea at night was at 6 o'clock and nearly always consisted of salad. On weekends in winter we'd have Mum's vegetable soup, but once again followed by salad. We did have cooking day on Saturday to bake cakes and slices or cookies for the Sunday family outing which was often a picnic.

As a family with six children mum was on a tight budget so when meat was served up, each of us would have a small portion as an accompaniment to a plate full of our vegies. The fruit and vegetables were free, they came from the back garden so we only ate what was in season. I still remember the day in winter that Mum came home from shopping at the local general store. She was incredibly impressed, there were fresh tomatoes to buy. Tomatoes weren't in season - where on earth would they have found those?!!

29

As for the vegetables, any that us kids wouldn't eat cooked, Mum put aside as she was preparing dinner and we'd go away munching them raw. We loved raw carrot, raw cabbage, raw beans, raw peas - a real delicacy, sweet and juicy, or raw turnip or swede/rutabaga (the only way to eat turnip!), all straight from Dad's garden. Mum figured that so long as we ate them cooked or raw we'd still be getting full nutritional benefit from them. Little did she realise that she was setting the example for the rest of my life.

Back then, life and food were simple. *We weren't living to eat, we were eating to live*. Diseases - asthma, heart disease, atherosclerosis / arteriosclerosis, diabetes, osteoporosis - were not in epidemic proportions as they are today. As a matter of fact, some of these diseases we had never heard of, so what are we eating today that we didn't in the past? Every way we turn we see influential advertisements 'drink milk - eat dairy foods' with the threat of crumbling bones, broken hips, rotting teeth ... The Dairy Industry has run a very efficient and effective advertising campaign even convincing our doctors, nutritionists and dietitians. But perhaps we'd better look at some real hard facts.

To begin with, countries with the highest consumption of dairy foods, USA, Australia, Sweden, Finland, have the greatest incidence of osteoporosis! In countries such as Japan, China and across Asia osteoporosis is almost unknown and dairy food is not a natural part of their diet. Have you ever wondered about the African children we see on TV being 'saved' from starvation by us, the Western World, with our generous donation of our glut of powdered milk? They're being given milk because we say they need it for nutrition but they can't digest it. It merely results in their noses running with mucous to their lip. It's totally foreign to their bodies. Africa's natives have a lower tolerance to dairy foods, even more than the rest of the world's population.

If you analyse Mother's Milk, for every 100gms it contains just 33 milligrams of calcium specially designed for human bones. Cow's milk is loaded with calcium and a very high amount of protein, and as pointed out by Robert Cohen, Director of the Dairy Education

Board in USA, " Baby humans don't grow up to become 550kg/1000lb cows". I quote the *Oxford Medical Dictionary* on its definition of milk which supports what I know. *Milk n. the liquid food secreted by female mammals from the mammary gland. It is the sole source of **food for the young of most mammals at the start of life**. Milk is a complete food in that it has most of the nutrients necessary for life: protein, carbohydrate, fat, minerals, and vitamins. The composition of milk varies very much from mammal to mammal. Cow's milk contains nearly all the essential nutrients but is comparatively deficient in vitamins C and D. Human milk contains more sugar (lactose) and less protein than cows' milk.*

Cows themselves don't drink milk, but obtain their calcium from plant based foods, as Mother Nature intended for us. Once we're adults our bones are already formed and no amount of extra calcium is going to strengthen them. We've become obsessed with the need for calcium, but our bones and bodies are not made of just calcium. It's also vital that our bodies take in the mineral magnesium for the absorption of calcium along with a good supply of vitamin D manufactured in our bodies from sunshine. Excess calcium deposits itself in different parts of the body causing painful arthritis (calcium crystals in the joints wearing them away). It can cause kidney stones (advertisement on the radio this very morning - 60 people a day are admitted to hospital in Australia with kidney stones), gall stones, and calcium buildup on the walls of arteries resulting in atherosclerotic plaques. It's also suspected of causing breast cancer and prostate cancer. This is just the tip of the iceberg.

Once again, to quote the words of Robert Cohen, "Osteoporosis is not a problem that should be associated with a lack of calcium intake. Osteoporosis results from calcium loss." The consumption of large amounts of protein in milk and animal protein results in a loss of calcium from the body. It's gleaned from the bones, filtered through into the bloodstream and passed out through the kidneys.

Calcium is more readily utilised by the body when it is obtained from plants. As I've already mentioned, combined with other necessary vitamins and minerals, especially magnesium, absorption aided by vitamin D, which in turn is manufactured in our body with the aid of the sun. All our green leafy vegetables, nuts, particularly raw almonds (one of the richest sources), cabbage, parsley, carrots and other root vegetables contain readily absorbable amounts of calcium, magnesium and essential minerals required for its assimilation. Regular exercise such as walking is very important in maintaining strong healthy bones. As the saying goes, "Use it or lose it."

Another factor in calcium loss is the consumption of excess salt. "I don't eat much salt" you might say, but if you read the ingredients on packet and tinned/canned foods you buy from the supermarket you'll find large amounts of salt by many different names - salt, sodium, sodium iodide, sodium chloride, potassium chloride, mineral salt, MSG, flavor enhancer and the list goes on. Calcium dissolves in the presence of sodium, passes into the bloodstream and out via the kidneys.

Coffee intake, alcohol and steroid medication are other causes of calcium loss. And it's not just restricted to women, men can also suffer from calcium deficiency.

This is only a very brief summary of the calcium debate. For much more information you can start by accessing www.notmilk.com Australia, USA or UK on the internet and find some of the research done in other parts of the world. You'll discover such headings as -

"Milk: Is the White Stuff the Right Stuff?
It was just six thousand years ago that the first settled communities, with their new found genius for growing crops and domesticating animals..."

"Osteoporosis - The Myths
Osteoporosis - The Bones of Contention to the medical hype, synthetic hormonal drugs, dairy products and most calcium supplements actually weaken the bones and have other harmful effects on health..."

You will find a long list of health problems from the consumption of dairy foods. It   can cause iron deficiency in infants, causes chronic constipation, Type 1 Diabetes (juvenile diabetes due to a type of protein in the milk which causes an autoimmune reaction); colicky babies, ovarian cancer, cataracts. It's been linked to childhood leukemia. All this I can believe because we live in a large, famous dairying area and I can quote names of a number of children and adults in our area with these diseases, in particular childhood diabetes, and three small children with leukemia. Go investigate these web sites and read for yourself, and you be the judge.

The Cholesterol Myth

Still on the subject of milk we look at one simple process that does much damage - homogenisation.
Homogenisation is the splitting up of the fat globules in milk so that they become evenly dispersed throughout. All that this process accomplishes is the prevention of cream from rising to the top of the milk. One has to wonder what relevance this natural occurrence has to preserving our health and wellbeing, especially once you've read the following explanation I've uncovered in some research.

The split fat globules after homogenisation are minute and have very sharp edges. Our body doesn't recognise these tiny molecules so they pass through undigested into the blood stream where they bump into and abrade arterial walls. This action causes a protective reaction and the body produces cholesterol to line the arterial walls, to protect them from the irritation caused by the sharp fat globules. Hence you have atherosclerosis. The high amount of cholesterol found in the blood by the doctor is really the body's protective mechanism springing into action. The doctor in his ignorance prescribes cholesterol - lowering drugs but with what side effects, remembering that it's an unnatural substance with which they're assaulting our bodies? As my husband Geoff loves to say, "for every action there is a reaction". So what kind of reaction does it cause in us?

Our English friends Phil and Penny Wheater recently sent us a book by biologist, Dr Robin Baker called *Fragile Science - The Reality Behind the Headlines*. In this book Robin Baker puts forward some valid points on a number of very controversial topics including 'What if Sunscreens Cause Skin Cancer?', 'Cholesterol: The Good, the Bad and the Ugly' and 'Clinical Depression and the House of Cards'. He makes you think and want to ask questions of medical scientists. What if cholesterol is an important protective mechanism in our body? What happens to us when cholesterol is artificially lowered by drugs? Apart from the side effect of the drug…!

In Dr Baker's words, "Cholesterol is an important chemical in the human body. It is vital for the healthy membrane structure of cells, for fertility and for embryonic development; pregnant rats given drugs that block the manufacture of cholesterol produce deformed foetuses. It is also involved in the production of hormones and bile - and probably in many more biochemical pathways still unknown."

Another quote from *'Fragile Science'*, Dr Baker states that "More than forty trials - involving well over 100,000 people - have now tested whether the deliberate lowering of cholesterol levels - by diet or by drugs - prevents heart attacks. In some trials the number of fatal heart attacks was lowered a little, but in others they actually increased … In fact, the number of deaths from all causes seemed to go up - from 5.8% to 6.1% - suggesting that high cholesterol may even have a protective role against some life-threatening factors." It makes you think doesn't it?

The last days of my mother's life were spent trying to adhere to a strict diet because her doctor told her that her cholesterol was up, and her blood pressure was very high. She said to me not long before she died, "How much less can I eat and nothing is working." She died a short time afterwards from a cerebral haemorrhage. At the time one of the doctors in attendance at the hospital stated that the blood pressure medication she'd been on for a number of years was known to cause a weakening of arterial walls. Was her cholesterol trying to protect her? It was around this time I started to ask lots of questions of my own.

If only I'd known then what I know now. A total change of her diet to our ***primitive diet*** I know would have solved Mum's health problems.

To some degree I feel her health could have been a little bit my fault. My husband Geoff had become a cheese maker and I was keeping Mum in cheese, a food that she had rarely fed us while we were growing up. But I also have to remember that it was the way I lost her that began our change in life. Incidentally, I had my cholesterol checked some time ago out of curiosity. I had a cholesterol level of 3. Perhaps it's our healthy raw food?

See if you can obtain a copy of Dr Baker's book, although I don't agree with all of his lines of reasoning. One chapter 'GM Foods: Monstrous Saviours' we disagree with strongly. How arrogant are we that we think we can improve on Nature? However, he does get you thinking on all topics.

If you access *The Cholesterol Myth* on the internet you'll find much scientific research on the effects of cholesterol also.

Do your own research, visit libraries, check the internet, and use your commonsense. Commonsense tells me that just because our body is out of balance it doesn't call for an attack by foreign, toxic substances to fix the problem. Our food and herbs should be our medicine.

Asthma

One of the many articles on diet and food that I've read recently summed it up perfectly – 'Nature's perfect food for baby cows is most certainly not Nature's perfect food for human beings.'

Three-quarters of the population of planet Earth cannot tolerate cow's milk. Casein, the protein in milk, is the most allergenic of all bovine proteins. Casein represents 80% of all milk protein, it's also the glue used to adhere labels to bottles and the glue used to hold wood together. Before his death, Dr Benjamin Spock, world renowned childhood expert declared casein, the milk and cheese protein, to be the cause of most allergies such as asthma, skin problems and digestive problems in babies and children and also the main reason for juvenile or Type 1 Diabetes in children. Because of the body's inability to digest casein, it passes through into the bloodstream and is transported to the organs of the body acting as glue, congesting and inflaming lungs and airways.

Add to this the intolerance of humans to lactose, the sugar in milk and milk's acidic affect on the body, and we can see the reason for the escalation of asthma, diabetes, gastrointestinal problems and other illnesses in our population as we are constantly urged to drink and eat 'dairy'.

Eczema

Eczema is an inflammation of the skin. It itches and can appear as a rash, weeping blisters, dry scaly patches of skin that is sometimes hardened, and in more severe cases, cracked. Eczema is mostly found inside of elbows, knees, wrists and patches can be found on the face.

Eczema frequently accompanies asthma and while it's believed that they are hereditary diseases, the genetic weakness may exist, but it's really the diet that is hereditary. Many sufferers of asthma and eczema also develop hayfever.

Once again we must relate back to our diet and the eating of foods that we're not meant to eat. Dairy is a major culprit in all these illnesses. If we eliminate the dairy, the grain, red meat and processed foods, then replace them with fresh fruits and vegetables rich in vital vitamins and minerals, add fresh fish, cold pressed oils, organic eggs and raw nuts and we should see an improvement. We need to eat fresh raw cabbage to cleanse our digestive system, raw carrot for Vitamin A, to boost our low immune system, lots of fresh raw greens and go out into the purifying, health giving sunshine - it's free!

I always suspect *Candidiasis* is running rife through the body causing poor digestion, so sugar and all processed foods should be left out. If conventional medicines have been used then this would definitely be the case, since cortisone ointment is one of the common applications, and any internal drugs taken will totally upset the body's balance.

For a good cleansing and immune boost, refer to the fresh, raw food guidelines I have mentioned for *Psoriasis*.

Supplements

- Ester C powder
- Vitamin A
- Vitamin E
- Zinc - many of us are deficient in zinc.
- Cod liver oil or fish oil
- I would definitely take echinacea for an immune boost
- Liver tonic to give a helping hand to eliminate toxins
- Digestive enzymes to aid in digestion

Remember, these supplements won't be necessary forever, just until your body is coping and achieving a healthy balance.

Diabetes

The consumption of dairy products has been linked to Insulin Dependant Diabetes Mellitus, or Type 1 Diabetes in children. Recent studies have shown a relationship between early exposure of babies to bovine proteins and the onset of diabetes.
Following recent studies on the rate of diabetes in Finland, USA and Japan it was found that the country with the highest milk and cheese consumption, Finland, had the highest rate of Type 1 Diabetes, 28 to every 100,000 per population. USA was next with 15, and Japan came a very low 1. (Report from *Lancet* 1992 : Greene et.al) It was believed that diabetes was hereditary but another report appearing in the *American Journal of Clinical Nutrition*, 1990 by FW Scott showed escalation of diabetes rates after native born Polynesians moved to Australia and changed their diets from fish proteins to cow proteins.

Scientific American (October 1992) declared The National Dairy Board's slogan 'Milk.- It does a body good', sounds a little hollow these days. It referred to evidence a team of Canadian researchers had discovered that early exposure of babies to cow's milk sometimes leads to diabetes. October 1996 in the *Lancet* it was written that antibodies to beta-casein are present in over one third of Type 1 Diabetes and almost non-existent in healthy individuals.

December 14, 1996 in *Lancet* Simon Murch MD of the Department of Paediatric Gastroenterology of the Royal Free Hospital, London wrote: "Cow's milk proteins are unique in one respect: in industrialized countries they are the first foreign proteins entering the infant gut, since most formulations for babies are cow milk-based. The first pilot study of our IDD prevention study found that oral exposure to dairy milk proteins in infancy resulted in both cellular and immune response... this suggests the possible importance of the gut immune system to the pathogenesis of IDD." Our body is continuously manufacturing new cells. We grow new hair, nails, lung and blood cells and of coarse new pancreatic beta cells - those required for production of insulin.

It was reported many years ago that Dr Albert Schweitzer suffered from severe diabetes. Following consultation with Max Gerson, one of the raw food promoters of the day, Dr Schweitzer was weaned from his high protein diet and on to a diet of raw vegetables and fruits, and especially fresh juices. Within a short period of time Dr Schweitzer was no longer insulin dependent, he was cured of his diabetes and lived to the wonderful old age of 90.

To sum it all up, we're told to eat dairy to prevent or slow down osteoporosis. Our doctors freely hand out cholesterol controlling pills (with untold side effects) and we're put on cholesterol free diets. We have puffers from which to inhale to free our airways (containing some very deadly chemicals and hormones) and we're told to reduce our sugar intake to prevent diabetes and here you are, here's some insulin to help you along -

but, since taking all these measures for our health why have these diseases escalated and reached epidemic proportions?

Candidiasis

What is it ?

Candida albicans is one of many yeasts naturally occurring in the vagina and alimentary tract (digestive system) of the human body. Description from the *Oxford Medical Dictionary* - 'The species *C.Albicans*, a small oval budding fungus, is primarily responsible for *candidosis'* (ie candidiasis). While the human body remains healthy these yeasts are kept in control by the body's main line of defence, the immune system, but because of today's diet, lifestyle, environment and use of drugs the immune system quickly becomes overpowered.

The *candida* yeast is mainly found in the gastrointestinal and genitourinary tracts kept in control by friendly bacteria such as lactobacillus acidophilus and bifidus. These helpful, friendly bacteria as well as being good 'bullies', produce one of the B group vitamins, Biotin which acts as an inhibitor on the yeast. Unfortunately, once the body has encountered our modern food, stress, drugs and environment the balance is upset, the 'goodies' are killed off and opportunist *Candida albican* yeast begins to rampantly grow.

Here I will explain my understanding of this yeast. It's neither a virus nor bacteria but a small plant with 'roots'. When the balance of the body is upset and the friendly bacteria are killed off it allows the roots of the *Candida* to penetrate the gut lining and grow. Once these roots penetrate the gut wall undigested proteins are able to pass through into the blood stream. Our body sees these as foreign and potentially dangerous, and produces antibodies to try to fight them, thus causing allergic reactions. The yeast cells colonise the surface of our mucous membranes and send their roots searching for food while at the same time producing toxins. The toxins enter the blood stream and circulate to every extremity of our body.

Main causes

- the suppression of the immune system as noted below and our obsession for cooked, processed, unnatural foods which feed the *Candida* yeast, allowing it to growth.

- antibiotic use - believed to be the greatest cause
- oral contraceptives
- hormone replacement therapy
- steroids, corticosteroids (cortisone or predinsone)
- inhalants for treatment of *asthma*
- anti-ulcer medication
- impaired liver function from chemical damage, including pesticides, herbicides and fungicides
- weakened immune system due to cancer treatments eg chemotherapy, radiation; environmental chemicals, *hypothyroidism, diabetes*, alcohol
- major stress
- antibiotics in the food chain eg chicken meat, beef, dairy food
- intake of other chemicals in foods eg sulphur as a preservative in wines

Symptoms
- thrush - vaginal yeast infection
- *Cystitis* - (bladder infection)
- skin problems - *Acne, Urticaria (hives), Psoriasis*, fungal infections such as T*inea pedis* (athlete's foot), fungal infections of the nails, fungal infections in the groin (jock itch) or beneath the breasts (red itchy rash), skin rashes, *Eczema*
- headaches, muscle aches and/or weakness, pain and/or swelling in and around the joints, uncoordination
- mental problems - mental fatigue, mental confusion, forgetfulness, inability to concentrate, mood swings, irritability, depression, manic depression, *Schizophrenia*
- gastrointestinal problems - bloating, gas, intestinal cramps, constipation, *Diarrhoea*, thrush in the mouth (especially babies), rectal itching
- infantile colic
- itchy nose, ears, eyes, anus
- allergies
- chemical sensitivities especially to the smell of perfumes, soaps, household cleaning products and petrochemicals, insect sprays
- cravings for yeast and sugar rich foods such as breads, cheese,

biscuits, chocolate, alcohol or vinegar
- a general unwell feeling in damp weather or in damp conditions as in caves, cellars or the garden
- just generally unwell for no apparent reason

Other associated conditions
- *Irritable Bowel Syndrome*
- *sensitivity to foods*
- menstrual complaints, *Premenstrual Syndrome*
- *Endometriosis*
- *Prostatitis*
- *Psoriasis*

The symptoms seem endless, don't they? Lots of these symptoms I know well, having 'been there - done that' a lot of years ago. I went through so many attacks of *Cystitis*, then thrush from all the antibiotics, muscle weakness, joint pains, many serious bouts with hives, so serious that when the enormous welts joined up I would pass out each time I sat or stood. At the same time my face, hands or feet would swell. I suffered abdominal bloating and severe intestinal cramps the moment I ate a grain food. My body reacted as though I had a bowel blockage. My nose and ears would become very itchy and I continually used olive oil in my ears to relieve the itch. I'm very intolerant of chemicals still, especially because I now know what they do to us. My biggest problem is with women and their chemical perfumes and deodorants, and men with their after shave- lotions and deodorants containing formaldehyde and other petrochemicals chemicals. I have to politely back away, feeling sorry for these people that they are so ill-informed of the damage they're doing themselves. The chemicals in their toiletries are absorbed directly into their blood stream through the pores of their skin, doing untold damage.

At my lowest point of health I'd built up many food intolerances. Oranges, mandarins, peaches, nectarines, apricots and pineapple caused major painful *Cystitis-like* bouts but once I realised this, I left them out of my diet. Now I eat all these fruits again without the slightest reaction. Pineapples and apricots are important as part of our medicine foods. Minute amounts of dairy brought on serious bouts of hives, as did a spoonful of cream, a taste of yoghurt or a very small cube of cheese. We knew that dairy food was not for humans, but if we went visiting or to dinner it was near impossible to eat a meal without it being in there in some form.

According to the gynaecologist I was sent to in a Sydney clinic, I had also had *Endometriosis* but he was extremely puzzled. He couldn't understand how it had been cured merely leaving scars in evidence. After we left the clinic, Geoff and I had a chuckle about this…how does one tell the doctor that you live on fresh vegetable juices, no dairy (known to be a major causative factor in *Endometriosis*), no red meat and mostly raw food? To explain *Endometriosis* according to the *Oxford Medical Dictionary* - it's 'the presence of tissue similar to the lining of the uterus at other sites of the pelvis…The tissue may also be found in the ovary, Fallopian tubes, pelvic ligaments, on the pelvic peritoneum, and even in the cervix and the vagina. This tissue undergoes the periodic changes similar to those of the endometrium (mucous membrane lining the uterus) and causes pelvic pain and severe *Dysmenorrhoea* (the formation of pelvic adhesions, a common sequel to *Endometriosis*). In such circumstances the uterus, Fallopian tubes and ovaries may need to be surgically removed in order to alleviate the symptoms.'

In more recent times our daughter, Rebecca has had reason to do some research on *Endometriosis*. She found that the eating of dairy food was one of the main causes of this very painful problem. My personal belief is that it's closely associated with *Candida*. With our total change of diet, by eating mostly raw vegetables, fruit and nuts as well as daily intake of fresh vegetable juices, I had actually cured myself of *Endometriosis*.

I've learnt so much over these last 25 years. Experience has taught me that trial and error but mostly success, proves far more than all the scientific research and theories combined. I've read books. I've checked research undertaken in other parts of the world, often with important evidence and results that for some unknown reason has been hidden away from the public, but success stories of people curing themselves of different diseases, have been a priority. ***They are the proof.***

Then there are the stories of long-lived old civilisations. They must have been doing something right, they never suffered these diseases and as with the Hunzas, lived life well beyond 120 years of age, peacefully going to sleep and never waking when their time had come. How long since you've heard of a healthy elderly friend or relative passing away peacefully from this life?

The author of my second health 'bible' that I talk of is Dr Patrick Kingsley. He was a doctor way ahead of his time. It was his experience as a clinical ecologist that proved to me that we were on the right path to solving the problem of *Candida albicans* and other major health problems. He firmly believed that the overgrowth of *Candida* yeast is the cause of around 90% of today's modern diseases, *Candida* and allergies to foods that are not natural to the human diet eg milk and grain. I don't need convincing of this either. Geoff and I have become people watchers. By a quick look at the eyes, the face, then the shape of people, and we can tell how ill they are and what many of their health problems are. Because I'm so sensitive to many smells I can detect the *Candida* yeast on the skin of a lot of people, mostly men who believe that they are tough and healthy. A glance in their eyes or at their faces usually tells a different story. So, as I keep preaching, take responsibility for your own health.

Essential foods
Here I disagree a little with the naturopaths and other alternate health practitioners, but then they speak from the benefit of their study, I speak only from the benefit of my experience of my very lowest time due to *Candida*. When I asked our daughter, Rebecca to write this chapter she told me that it would be better coming from me with my personal battle with it. We've had friendly discussions and I've learnt a lot from her, and we've had disagreements over certain aspects, her views being that of a naturopath. To Rebecca's credit, a number of times she's gone away, thought about it and come back later to graciously declare that what I've said had merit.

43

I totally agree that sugars have to be omitted from the diet - sugar processed from sugar cane, sugar beet, rice syrup, malt, honey and maple syrup. I tend to disagree with the theory that the naturally occurring sugar, fructose found in fresh raw fruit can cause *Candida* to grow. In the years of my gradual recovery I found that if I didn't eat fruit I became very lethargic and my bowel didn't operate well. Then I asked myself "Would this fresh fruit sugar feed yeast to make the bread rise?" As we used to make our own bread I couldn't see this happening, so I went back to having fruit and still suffer no consequences. You be your own judge, if you feel you've had an adverse reaction to a fruit or fruits, try omitting it for a week or two then try it again. A reaction can take from minutes to a couple of days to show.

Both a dietitian and a naturopath in the early days told me that I should eat mainly cooked food, that too much raw food was no good for me as it was harsh on my digestion. Against my better judgement I was an obedient patient and I went back to eating more cooked food and suffered a similar result as with omitting fresh fruit. I was tired, my body was 'blocked up' and I began putting on weight, to my mind because it was blocked with unnatural, dead food. I happily went back to my raw food.

I totally agree that we shouldn't drink alcohol in any shape or form. Vinegars are in this category also. The making of alcohol and vinegar relies on fermentation, the growing of yeasts and moulds, addition of sugars and malts and chemicals as well. I know you won't like me saying so, but I, too was a little partial to wines once, in particular good champagne. If now we're out for a very special occasion I will have a glass but for the few days following, it leaves me very washed out and 'brain dead'. I think medical practitioners are extremely irresponsible to promote wine as being healthy for us, especially the effect it has on the liver. Vinegars I consider to be worse. If you check *The Oxford Dictionary* you'll find vinegar described as 'sour liquid (diluted acetic acid) produced by acetous fermentation of wine'). If you want the lining of your digestive tract stripped then use vinegar. White vinegar is most suited to household cleaning chores! These are the reasons for replacing vinegars in mayonnaise and dressings with fresh lemon, lime or orange juice and you have the added bonus of Vitamin C.

I disagree with alternate health practitioners when they say that we shouldn't eat organic, sulphur-free dried fruits. One of the reasons given for omitting these fruits is that when the fruit is picked for drying it can carry yeasts and moulds. Just once or twice I've been aware of a mouldy sultana but they were conventionally grown not organic. The other reason is the fructose, fruit sugar content. Apart from that we dry fruits in our solar drier, and purchase dried figs, nectarines, dates, sultanas, raisins and currants as a major part of our diet. I've never suffered an adverse reaction to them. Organic dried figs and apricots are rich in iron and other essential nutrients. This plant-based iron is far more readily digested and utilised by our body than that of meat so it makes them important in balancing our diet.

I agree that mushrooms and other fungi should only be eaten as a special treat but you be the judge of that for yourself. As for any other food, if you notice they have a reaction with you, then leave them out of your diet.

And, of course, dairy food, especially cheese, should be eradicated from your diet. The older, more mature a cheese is, the worse it is. Then we should remember that milk can contain traces of antibiotics or other chemicals if a cow has been suffering from illness such as mastitis, and that the milk has been pasteurised which kills any live enzyme that might have been the slightest bit helpful to our wellbeing. Final point and perhaps the main point on dairy food ... it all should be avoided due to its being a major allergen. All allergens need to be eliminated from the diet since allergies weaken our immune system making conditions favourable for the growing of the *Candida yeast*.

The main aim is to starve the *Candida yeast* and boost the immune system to give it the power to do its job. Part of this is restoring and maintaining a healthy liver to allow it to carry out one of its main tasks, that of filtering chemicals and toxins from our blood.

So, eat organic carrots, cabbage, spinach/silverbeet, lettuces, beetroot, celery, garlic, ginger; parsley, thyme, sage, rosemary (add these herbs chopped fresh to your salads, they have antifungal properties), apples, paw paw/papaya, grapefruit and bananas, then all the rest of your fresh vegetables and fruits. Nuts - the most important is the almond, then pine nuts, pecans, and don't forget our very own macadamia nut, add a mixture of the others and you're not doing too bad! Dried fruits such as organic figs, apricots and dates particularly for their iron content.

Fresh vegetable juices with the addition of garlic and ginger should be taken atleast twice a day. Garlic and ginger with their powerful antifungal properties are simple, cheap, natural medicines

Keep following *A Primitive Diet* with lots of organic raw vegetables, fruits and nuts. Don't forget herbs as your medicine ... and read your body. It will tell you if something upsets it.

Supplements
- *Lactobacillus acidophilus* and *bifidus* (dairy free) to replace this friendly bacteria already killed off in the intestines
- Ester C powder (from health food stores)
- Flaxseed oil
- Caprylic acid - a naturally occurring fatty acid known to be effective against the *Candida* yeast
- digestive enzymes - to aid in the absorption of nutrients from your food
- liquid liver tonic - to get the liver operating at optimum level
- slippery elm powder - heaped teaspoon before bed each night; it lines and soothes the digestive tract while at the same time prevents the *Candida* from attaching to the intestinal wall. I cheat a little when taking slippery elm powder. Because it's so tasteless I mix it in a small amount of juice, add boiling water then I quickly drink it down before it turns too gluggy!
- multi-vitamin and mineral supplement (sugar-free, yeast-free, dairy-free, check label)
- zinc
- selenium
- biotin - a type of B vitamin which acts to kill off the *Candida* yeast

These supplements are those recommended by Dr Kingsley and the

Encyclopaedia of Natural Medicine. Through the taking of these natural medicines I've pulled myself up to be as well as I am today. If you're not confident in helping yourself there are many excellent naturopaths around who are only too willing to give you a hand.

You might think all the above supplements seem a lot to take but remember that your body has probably been out of balance for a long time and it needs a helping hand to be restored to optimum health. As you improve, some of these can be phased out. The aim is to get your liver well and doing its job of filtering the toxins from your blood. You need your immune system up and fighting and your digestion operating correctly so that the nutrients can be absorbed from your food. People become very defensive when you say they have a malabsorption problem. They say they only eat good food, but if their digestion is not working as it should, which is most of us, then our nutrients pass through our body without being absorbed.

This is my understanding of *Candida*. I do hope it helps you in some way. If you want to know more check on the Internet, go to your local library, your local book store, the information is there. Then, do as I do, give thought to what sounds like commonsense and what doesn't. I do know that the lifestyle we've lived all these years has benefited us greatly and I sometimes wonder what the result would have been had I persevered with conventional medicine.

Coeliac Disease

What is it ?

Coeliac disease is a condition where the villi and absorptive cells of the small intestines are damaged or destroyed, impairing digestion and the absorption of vital nutrients. It is caused by a reaction to the protein *gliadin*, a component of gluten that is found in the grains wheat, spelt, rye, barley, millet, triticale and oats. In persons with coeliac disease the gliadin portion of gluten causes an abnormal immune response in the mucus lining of the intestine. The inflammation and damage to the absorptive cells causes malabsorption and malnourishment.

Symptoms

- diarrhoea,
- cramps
- flatulence
- nausea
- vomiting
- bloating
- poor appetite
- abdominal distention
- abdominal pain
- mouth ulcers
- pale, frothy, foul-smelling, greasy stools with increased faecal fat
- weakness
- weight loss and multiple vitamin and mineral deficiencies

- muscle wasting
- irritability, depression
- fatigue
- stunted bulky growth
- intense burning sensation in the skin
- red, itchy skin rash (dermatitis herpetiformis)

Note. Gut symptoms need not be present. The disease may manifest as eczema, arthritis, mouth ulcers and kidney disease.

The effects of *Coeliac Disease* are usually reversed after the removal of all gluten from the diet.

Avoid all foods containing gluten
wheat, rye, triticale, spelt, oats, barley, millet
commercial foods that have wheat or gluten components.

Watch for hidden sources of gluten
- beer, wine, vodka, whiskey
- natural flavours
- hydrolysed vegetable protein
- textured vegetable protein (TVP)
- hydrolysed plant protein
- luncheon meat, sausages
- gravies (Gravox)
- mustard, curry powder, seasonings
- 'wheaten' cornflour
- modified food starch
- malt
- soy sauce
- tomato sauce, ketchup
- white vinegar, grain vinegars
- soup
- ice cream

Note. Dairy products should be avoided and all food allergens should be determined and eliminated.

It should be mentioned here to watch for any adverse reactions to eating buckwheat, a common replacement for wheat. After I'd had reactions to eating it a number of times a check revealed that buckwheat actually has a type of protein very similar to gluten.

Coeliac Facts
- A zinc deficiency may contribute to *Coeliac Disease*. The condition will be unresponsive to dietary therapy if an underlying zinc deficiency is present.

- Milk intolerance is a contributing factor in *Coeliac Disease*.
- Lactose intolerance can occur with *Coeliac Disease*.
- Breastfeeding has been shown to have a preventative effect as breastfed babies have a decreased risk of developing *Coeliac Disease*.
- *Coeliac* symptoms commonly appear in the first three years of life and the early introduction of cereal grains and cow's milk are believed to be major causative factors.
- *Coeliac Disease* may be hereditary. Factors that may trigger the onset of the disease are emotional stress, intestinal infection, viral infection, physical trauma, pregnancy or surgery.
- A deficiency of the digestive enzymes involved in protein digestion may contribute to *Coeliac Disease*.
- Epidemiological, clinical and experimental studies have suggested that wheat gluten components are a causative factor in the development of schizophrenia. Wheat gluten components have demonstrated opium-like activity.
- Conditions such as thyroid abnormalities, *Schizophrenia*, dermatitis (herpetiformis) and *Urticaria* (hives) have been linked to gluten intolerance.

Suggested Supplemental help for Coeliacs

- Digestive enzymes - to improve digestion;
- Essential fatty acids such as evening primrose oil, salmon oil supplements, and use cold pressed olive oil in salad dressings. They're needed for the villi in the intestines and as an anti-inflammatory;
- Aloe vera juice - healing to the gut lining and aids digestion;
- Slippery elm - soothes and heals the gut mucosa and is a nutritious agent in a sensitive digestive system;
- Zinc Taste Test / supplement - check for zinc deficiency and supplement if necessary;
- High potency multi-vitamin and mineral complex - to correct nutritional deficiencies and prevent further deficiencies due to malabsorption;
- Folic acid - necessary for the health and maintenance of the villi of the small intestine and a deficiency can cause the *Coeliac* symptoms;

- Vitamin A - deficiency is associated with *Coeliac Disease* and a vitamin A deficiency may be associated with a lack of zinc;
- Acidophilus and bifidus - aid digestion, enhance absorption of nutrients, inhibit disease-causing organisms, help detoxify harmful substances, and help manufacture B-complex vitamins and vitamin K.

Other herbs to consider
- Turmeric and ginger - anti-inflammatories;
- Liquorice root, marshmallow root - soothing and healing;
- Fenugreek seeds - healing, anti-inflammatory, nutritive, and tones digestive function.

Written by Rebecca Southam
Bach of Health Science (Complementary Medicine)
Dip. Naturopathy, Dip. Botanical Medicine, Dip. Nutrition

It's important to note here that <u>once</u> you have adjusted to your new diet, which can take some time, you have your illness in hand and you are in good health again not all these supplements are necessary; that is…as long as you eat wholesome, predominantly raw, organic nuts, fruits and vegetables that contain all their nutrients, and you are <u>digesting</u> them.

Lots of fresh raw foods aid in digestion. Paw paw/papaya contains the enzyme papain, which aids in the digestion of proteins. Then there is grapefruit, doctors warn that it's not good for you to eat because it makes prescription drugs (should you be on them) double their potency, so imagine their ability to help you with digestion of other foods. Pears are said to also aid digestion. Folic acid comes from green leafy vegetables, so eat lots of lettuces, cabbage, spinach/silverbeet, parsley, celery and especially broccoli. Vitamin A and beta carotene can be found in all the delicious orange and red fruits and vegetables such as carrots, with some eggs in there to make the vitamin complete. Get lots of good healthy sunshine, one of Nature's medicines and the source of Vitamin D that in turn works with calcium and magnesium to keep our bones healthy.

Ulcerative Colitis/Crohn's Disease and Irritable Bowel Syndrome

Ulcerative Colitis

Ulcerative Colitis is a chronic disorder affecting the mucous membranes lining the colon causing it to become inflamed and ulcerated. A person with this problem can experience gas, bloating, pain, diarrhea and even the passing of blood. This condition can develop into a severe illness with doctors suggesting removal of the lower colon and replacement with a colostomy bag. *This is not necessary!*

Crohn's Disease

Crohn's Disease is a condition of the alimentary tract (or digestive tract). As with ulcerative colitis it becomes inflamed and ulcerated, and can cause fever, headaches, malabsorption, chronic diarrhea, abdominal pain, even causing appendicitis like symptoms.

Irritable Bowel Syndrome

Irritable Bowel Syndrome, also called *Spastic Colon / Mucous Colitis*, is a condition causing abdominal pain, diarrhea or constipation, nausea, flatulence, bloating and food intolerances.

No matter what the diagnosis or the scientific approach with drugs, nothing works as effectively as using your food as your medicine, but before I outline the simple solution to these debilitating illnesses, I need to tell you David's story. I believe that the 'proof is in the pudding' and having also helped myself with bowel upsets due to *Candidiasis* I know how easy it is to heal the digestive tract.

I first spoke to David after meeting his daughter. She told me about her serious concerns for his health and could I please contact him. David had lost his wife in a tragic accident and undoubtedly the trauma and stress had upset his body's balance and immune system. He was diagnosed with ulcerative colitis and placed on medication. According to the specialist, the medication was to control the disease because there was no cure. The drugs befuddled his brain and made concentration difficult. He became worse and advised the specialist that the drugs weren't working, so the dose was doubled!

At the same time David was trying to keep up with his demanding job. He was experiencing interrupted sleep, rising to empty his bowel numerous times through the night, then working all day. By the end of his working day he was suffering from extreme exhaustion. He was desperately searching for answers because he wasn't improving, if anything his health was slipping further. He felt certain foods were causing a bad reaction but when he mentioned it to the specialist, the specialist told him food had nothing to do with it. The cause was unknown. During David's last visit, the specialist suggested the removal of his affected lower colon, to replace it with a colostomy bag. David was shocked. The specialist went on to tell him that he had friends who had colostomy bags, and they lived perfectly normal lives. David gave up on doctors and gave up on medication.

It was at this time that I met him. I told him about changing his diet because certain foods would be causing most of his problems. He was rather dubious but since he had already found that some foods did upset him, he was willing to try. I encountered the usual negative reaction when I told him no wheat, or grains containing gluten, no yeast, dairy foods, red meat, sugar, black tea and coffee, alcohol and vinegar. The very first comment *is* usually "what is there left to eat?" By taking away the 'bad' foods and his eating of more 'medicine' foods necessary for healing the digestive tract, David began to improve immensely. The next phone call I had from him he told me how he was sleeping through the night, and his energy was returning. Not long afterward, he headed off to visit his daughter overseas.

I spoke to David recently, after he returned home from a trip of some months that took him out working in Central Australia. He admitted that he isn't following his diet religiously but is more in control than when I met him early last year. Never was he going to slip back to the state in which he found himself not so long ago.

Main Medicine Foods

Carrots - eat raw, eat plenty and drink their juice. Carrots are a major medicine food, an important healer, immune booster and mucous eliminator.

Cabbage - eaten raw, along with carrots is the most essential vegetable for someone with digestive problems. Cabbage may cause a little wind in the first couple of days but in reality it's busy gently cleansing and healing the upset state of your digestive tract. Cabbage will clean out the debris clogging and putrefying the system, then work on the alkalinity to allow the digestive system to heal.

Apples - work in a similar way to cabbage. Apples will remineralise your body. The old saying "an apple a day keeps the doctor away" is a true statement. Eat for breakfast, lunch or dinner and/or last thing before bed at night. Occasionally I have felt a little bloating after eating apple if eaten on 'a cold stomach' mid morning. But, you can never eat too many.

Celery - is alkalising and cleansing. It contains the natural mineral salts necessary for healthy cells. Celery is also a natural healer and will help repair the damaged system and will prevent further toxic build up in the various parts of the body. An essential ingredient in your daily vegetable juice.

Garlic - a natural antibacterial, antifungal and antibiotic. We have one or two cloves in our vegetable juices twice daily as well as added to dressings. Don't be concerned about eating fresh garlic, it's not really noticeable on your breath.

Ginger - add a small piece to your vegetable juice. It's been known down through history as a superior treatment for soothing the gastrointestinal tract. It will settle the discomfort felt in a very short time. It's also warming and excellent for circulation, with antifungal and antibacterial properties. Make ginger tea by adding two or three slices to a cup and pour on boiling water. Allow to steep for a few minutes then sip.

Add to your diet fresh raw greens, lots of herbs, fresh fruit and vegetables, fresh organic eggs and organic chicken as a special treat from time to time. Purchase fresh fish. Try to purchase from local fishermen should you be so lucky to have ocean or lake nearby, this will help you avoid chemical contamination. Eat snacks of raw nuts and organic dried fruits. Leave out peanuts, these are legumes not nuts and are very acidic on the system.

Drink fresh herbal teas. Buy fresh herbs or grow them in pots or your flower garden. Take some leaves, add to the teapot or cup and pour on boiling water. Leave to stand for 5 - 6 minutes and you will have a healthy, refreshing drink. Try some catnip, lemon balm, lemon verbena and lemon grass to make a very nice lemon tea. The leaves of sage, thyme and rosemary form a powerful healing tea.

Basically, follow our *Primitive Diet* and you will find yourself eating your way to a long and healthy life.

Some suggested supplements

- Slippery elm powder - to soothe and heal.
- Ester C powder - to boost the immune system
- Liver tonic - to cleanse the liver of toxins and allow it to get on with its job
- Digestive enzymes - to help digest food and aid absorption of nutrients
- Echinacea - to boost the immune system
- Multivitamin and mineral supplement

Psoriasis

Psoriasis is a common chronic inflammation of the skin mostly involving the scalp, backs of knees, elbows and wrists and appears on the body as a red scaly rash. Since we are what we eat, we must look to our food first then our digestive system and immune system.

Our skin is the largest organ of our body and an unhealthy skin is an indication of impaired liver function, faulty digestion and a diet of food not meant for us. If our liver is over loaded with toxins or not functioning efficiently, then it can't filter the waste products from our blood through our bowel, especially if the wastes have passed through into our blood stream due to poor digestion. These wastes need to come out somewhere so they come out through the skin.

Conventional medicine's prescribing of cortisone-based creams and antibiotics merely aggravate the condition and add to the body's imbalance. There is a simple a solution to help yourself recover from the affects of psoriasis. Eliminate the bad unnecessary foods from your diet and replace with fresh fruits and vegetables, organic eggs and nuts with a good dose of purifying sunshine each day, and it's free!

To begin with, leave out all dairy food, gluten grains - wheat, rye, oats, barley, millet along with buckwheat, yeast, sugar, red meat, alcohol and limit coffee to no more than one a day if you must have it. These foods clog up and place a lot of pressure on our body's systems. For the good foods add lots more fresh, organic fruits and vegetables, especially these powerful medicine foods I'm about to mention.

Cabbage - first and foremost you need fresh, raw cabbage to sweep through your clogged digestive system including your bowel. The first day or two you may experience wind or bloating. It's the cabbage beginning to do its work.
Carrot - fresh and raw, particularly in the form of fresh juice, everyday. It provides necessary Vitamin A and is a major boost to the immune system.
Beetroot - raw, is a powerful liver tonic and cleanser so add a small

amount to your fresh carrot juice, or grate it into a salad.

Garlic - a natural antifungal, antibiotic, antibacterial and when added fresh to vegetable juice is not noticeable on the breath.

Spinach/silverbeet and other greens - for essential minerals, folic acid and chlorophyll.

Celery - contains natural salts necessary for the formation of healthy cells and to alkalise acid conditions. It also contains many essential minerals.

Apples - rich in minerals, is alkalising and cleansing like cabbage.

The remaining fresh fruit and vegetables are almost as important. Do limit eating potatoes, replace with sweet potato and parsnip. (Before potatoes were introduced to Europe from South America, parsnips were a staple of the European diet.)

Do have lots of vegetable juices. Eat fish, a little organic chicken, definitely organic eggs and nuts (not peanuts). Fruit, with the exception of oranges, are essential.

Helpful Supplements

- Ester C powder to build a healthy immune system
- Cod liver oil
- Zinc - our soils, and hence our food, is said to be deficient in zinc. This mineral is necessary for healing.
- Echinacea to boost the immune system
- Digestive tonic to assist the digestive system to get back on track.
- Liver tonic to give the liver a helping hand to detox.

Remember that these aren't necessary forever, they are a tool to help bring your body back into balance but the good food should continue forever. Follow our *primitive diet* and you should experience a psoriasis-free life.

Acne

Acne is a very common skin problem affecting teenagers going through puberty and to a lesser degree, mature adults. I found it very interesting that until my sisters, brothers and I were going through puberty and developed a rare pimple, my mother hadn't encountered *Acne*, or pimples as we called them. It was an extreme case, and it was rare to see someone with severe *Acne* as we do today. No doubt this is a sign of our unhealthy diet, fruits and vegetables lacking in their health giving nutrients, from growing in unhealthy soils, contaminated with artificial fertilisers and chemical sprays?

Acne is the most common skin disorder and is seen as pimples with a white head filled with pus, or it can be a blackhead, but mostly appearing on the face or to a lesser degree on the back. In its severest form it can cause terrible scarring of the skin. Conventional medicine believes that antibiotics will solve *Acne* but the alternate theory is, because the antibiotic causes an imbalance of the gut flora allowing *Candida yeast* to thrive, it can worsen the *Acne*.

Acne, like *Psoriasis* and *Eczema*, is easy to turn around. It is merely an indication of a clogged up, unbalance system and, with a good healthy diet with cleansing fresh foods, there is no reason not to be totally free of *Acne*. Please refer to the chapter on overcoming *Psoriasis* because, although all three skin disorders appear different, the reasons for being afflicted with them, and the way for overcoming them are the same. They are caused by similar allergies and intolerances, and is the skin indicating a faulty digestive system.

Follow our ***primitive diet*** and suggested food medicines for *Psoriasis,* and the suggested supplements (this is the course of action I would follow should I have these skin problems) and in no time your skin should begin to clear. Not only should your skin clear but it should reflect a healthy, more energetic you.

Multiple Sclerosis - a disease or not?

I have some special friends who haven't been as lucky in health as I, they have *Multiple Sclerosis*. It's been incredibly difficult to watch my friend, Susan, who possesses great artistic talent, quickly deteriorate from the effects of *Multiple Sclerosis*. Just a short time ago Susan was teaching me the joys of colour and design through silk painting but today she hoons around her house in a wheel chair trying to keep up with her son, Benjamin and husband, Brett.

After research into this terrible 'disease' I found it interesting that the geographical distribution of MS across the world is linked to countries and areas of high dairy and grain consumption, Canada, United States, Australia, New Zealand, Great Britain, northern Europe and Scandinavia. In Asian countries such as Japan and China, as well as in the so-called third world countries, it's rare or virtually unheard of. In our area around our town of Bega there is a large group of MS sufferers and of course Bega is a famous Australian dairying area.

The cause of MS has never been determined. Researchers are still groping in the dark trying to isolate a specific virus or viruses, but to date no positive results have been forthcoming to support this theory. Investigation into the thought that autoimmune factors could be involved has still proved nothing. Some researchers are still checking into the role diet might play in MS, comparing it with that of the Japanese people who consume a lot of seafood. Once again medical science is looking from the wrong angle. Why do they always look at the diet of races of people to see *what* they're eating? *Shouldn't they be looking to see what they don't eat?* I believe that 99% of medical solutions are under their noses.

When my friend Susan was first diagnosed I told her we would overcome it. Because of the way it was affecting her, I firmly believed it could be beaten by our diet and some supplements to get her body's digestive and immune systems back in operation, and in balance. I would like to mention here that my reason for this belief came from my own personal experience. Some time ago I discovered that if I ate grain which by now was foreign to me, my legs would become very heavy and it was quite difficult to walk up stairs, up hills, pretty much to walk at all. At the same time I would find myself suffering from a little incontinence, often barely making it to the toilet to pass urine. After a week or two once the toxic effects wore off I would return to normal again and I'd become my usual spritely self. Over a period of time I've discovered that even to have a treat of rice makes my legs heavy for a week or so.

Susan wasn't quite ready to accept this very simplistic idea. She frantically began her own research which took her round and round in circles many times. Anything she discovered she'd e-mail through to me so I could read it too. All I could do was be there anytime she wanted to talk about it, but I couldn't force my views on her. Recently I received a fantastic e-mail from her just saying to "click on the site below". Now, as I said, I'd received a number of e-mails from her over the last couple of years but most of them I read and thought them to be useless information. This time because I was busy writing I almost ignored it, put it aside to read it at a later date, but some sense willed me to click on it. Up came the story of Roger MacDougall. I sat and devoured every word on that screen as I scrolled through thirteen pages. At the end I threw my arms in the air cheering "YES, YES, YES!" There was the proof I needed that diet could overcome MS.

Roger's Story
Roger MacDougall was born in Scotland in 1910. He was a playwright, film writer, composer, songwriter and a musician. Roger wrote work for the Prince of Wales Theatre, London Palladium, BBC, British film studios plus many more so imagine the effect of such a devastating disease as MS on this talented man.

He was diagnosed in 1953 and quickly deteriorated until he found himself confined to a wheelchair. Not willing to accept that his condition was hopeless he began to search for information and study treatments of degenerative diseases till he decided to try a change of diet. Right here I feel that to do the story justice I need to quote Roger's own words straight from his book.

"I was now considering my body as a biochemical process, or, more accurately as a biochemical process going wrong. As I had not heard of allergy tests I had to find some other way of pinpointing the errors in my diet.

It seemed logical to stick to those foods which had been consumed by man since the very beginning. ***I based my diet on the food consumed by the hunter-gatherer, before mankind settled down in agricultural communities, grew cereals and tended cattle.***

It was this reasoning which led me to cut out gluten (a protein which surrounds the germ in grains), cow's milk and sugar. These are not foods from whose consumption we have evolved and I believe that the fact is in some way connected with our rejection of them. Not enough is known yet but the close connection between diet and illness becomes more and more obvious. When I removed my three principle allergens, I stopped deteriorating and eventually began to make slow but nonetheless steady improvement."

Roger began a diet of raw vegetables and fruit and their juices, free range animals - venison, rabbit and poultry with some liver, kidney, tongue (do watch the eating of offal though, these organs are the filters of toxic chemicals, eat organic as much as possible). He supplemented his diet with the vitamins and minerals that his body needed for his recovery.

Slowly he began to improve. In 1975 he revisited the neurologist at the National Hospital for Nervous Diseases in London, who had diagnosed his illness back in 1953. Thorough examination showed that his muscles, movement and reflexes were perfectly normal and the neurologist admitted that he'd never "encountered such a spectacular remission".

Roger MacDougall died just a few years ago, living well into his eighties, still totally free of MS, but to this day neurologists working with MS ignore his fantastic discovery and recovery.
After reading through his story I excitedly e-mailed Susan an "I told you

so" note. "So what are you waiting for girl? We have a date remember. We have Brown Mountain to climb the moment you're out of that wheelchair!" Brown Mountain is a steep rise of 1000 metres to the Southern Highlands behind our town of Bega. I made a date with Susan once, she told me that one day she was going to be well again and she was going to walk all the way to the top but we decided that she had to *push me up the mountain in her wheelchair.* That day I'm going to be out there shouting her success to the world.

Just a by-the-by here - I was talking to Sue afterwards to see how she was, and she'd been chuckling to a fellow MS sufferer "don't you just hate Bev, she was right all the time?!"

So…all you MS sufferers out there, get off your butts! You have to do it for yourself, no one can do it for you and no toxic chemical, magical drug or pill is going to solve it for you. ***And how simple is it?***

To access the website with the story of Roger MacDougall go into www.direct-ms.org/roger.html and read the abridged version written by A.F.Embry, or better still go to your local bookshop who should be able to order the full story in his book *My Fight Against Multiple Sclerosis.*. If your bookshop can't find a new copy then maybe they can get you a second hand copy.

Suggested Supplements
* Mega B vitamins (such as Tresos B)
* Selenium
* Ester C powder - ¼ teaspoon 2-3 times per day
* Vitamin E
* Magnesium / calcium
* Flaxseed oil - 1 tablespoon
* Cod liver oil - 1 tablespoon
* Heaped teaspoon slippery elm powder before bed

Raw organic fruits and vegetables I would especially eat daily
Cabbage - in salads, coleslaw, in vegetable juice

Carrots - grated and added to salads and coleslaw, as a base in vegetable juice
Beetroot - grated, added to salads, in vegetable juice (a liver cleanser)
Garlic - fresh, in juice, in dressings
Ginger – fresh, in juice
Apples - rich in minerals
Grapefruit - a digestive aid and alkalizing on the body
Paw paw/papaya - a digestive aid, a medicine fruit rich in vitamins and minerals
A good amount of lettuce and salad greens, parsley, spinach / silverbeet

Basically I would stick to the ***primitive diet*** in this book but I would leave out those special treats such as dampers, cakes, biscuits, rice and pastas that I've added due to special request. We don't see these as being necessary to our way of life but if you feel you have to have them, *remember to make sure the ingredients are organic.* I understand that after years of eating breads and other grain products, people feel there is something missing at their mealtime. These treats we tend to call 'comfort food'. Final word - Early Man wouldn't have eaten these foods either.

Autism and Immunisation

In conventional medical circles *Autism* is believed to be a brain or psychiatric disorder diagnosed in children around the age of three years. An autistic child can display indifference to their family and surroundings, they can withdraw into themselves, have difficulty speaking and communicating, learning, have behavioural problems and appear to have a low level of intelligence.

Conventional doctors treat autistic children with drugs to control their behavioural problems and suggest speech therapists to attempt to overcome speech difficulties. Then they will send you on your way because they're convinced there is nothing more that can be done. I'm about to tell you why I disagree with this whole way of thinking.

To begin with, it's well documented the damaging affects that immunisation has on babies, children and adults. In some realms of medicine it's known that immunisation is the major cause of *SIDS* (*Sudden Infant Death Syndrome*), *Autism, Hyperactivity, Arthritis, Asthma, HIV* and many more serious disorders. The supposed benefits of vaccinations have never been proven. We, and especially our innocent children, are the experiment.

Our babies are being injected with toxic chemicals within hours of being born. What are they injecting into our precious new born? It can be a whole chemical cocktail. According to Dr Joseph Mercola in the U.S.A. some of the additives include the preservative formaldehyde - a known carcinogenic; aluminium hydroxide - cancer producing; monosodium glutamate (MSG), we all know; phenoxyethanol – antifreeze. There can be animal tissues such as pig blood, horse blood, rabbit brain, dog or monkey kidney, chicken embryo, human diploid cells originating from aborted human foetal tissue. Then we have acetone we all know as nail polish remover; thimerosal - derived from mercury, a toxic heavy metal, and phenol (carbolic acid) - a deadly poison. The diseases such as polio and smallpox that immunisation are said to prevent had already almost disappeared right across the world by the time vaccinations came along. The World Health Organisation has admitted that their disappearance is due to the improved water supplies, sanitation, awareness of diet and nutrition, and better living conditions. It was not from immunisation. When I first undertook some research on this subject, the information left me stunned. The polio vaccine is actually the cause of the 3,000 reported cases of polio in the U.S. each year!

If you're fortunate to have access to a computer, please take time to research the devastating effects these have on our body. You'll find a lot more than I've told you here. Search for such articles as 'Tell the Truth About Vaccines - or Keep Away From My Children', 'Immunization. htm', *The Vaccine Guide* by Randall Neustaedter. It won't take much to convince you the course of action you need to take.

I was attending a health seminar a few months ago where parents were asking should they have their teenagers immunised against *Meningococcal.* The question was asked of the doctor in attendance, and the answer was cautiously given. Apart from the above mentioned preservatives, and the active ingredient of cultured bacteria or viruses, treated toxins or dead organisms, the way immunisations are administered proved conclusively to me that they are ineffectual.

Germs of most of the diseases regarded as 'killers' and 'maimers' are all around us. Many naturally occur on our skin, in air passages and gastrointestinal tract. Only when our immune system is weakened is there a remote chance of contracting any of these diseases. While the diseases and bacteria are mostly inhaled into the respiratory tract or swallowed, immunisations are injected into the blood stream, a totally different system. How can they act to protect us from disease? Rather I believe they weaken our immune system by the assault of toxic chemicals, viruses and bacteria directly into the blood stream, bypassing our natural defences that would come out fighting to kill them off immediately.

We are so naïve and trusting, especially with our precious babies, who are our future. But please don't feel guilty, many of us, me included, have believed and trusted our doctor. Don't get me wrong, we do need doctors to sew up and mend us following accidents. The rest of our ills and ails can be corrected by our diet and medicine foods, and herbs.

Now back to the problem of *Autism*. It's not a life sentence for your child, it's very simple to reverse. Let the natural food remove the toxins from your child's body. Take away the foods that aren't natural to us - dairy food, wheat and gluten grains, yeast and sugar. Immediately begin feeding fresh, raw, organic medicine foods such as carrot, cabbage and greens, lots of fruit, a little fish, no red meat and a treat of organic chicken once in a while. If a small child is given the choice of eating raw or cooked vegetables you will be very surprised to find that a child will choose raw. They haven't yet had their natural instincts tarnished by us. It's we adults who influence our children and tell them they don't like certain foods or raw foods. They learn by example.

Offer a plate of carrot and celery straws, small pieces of cabbage, little broccoli florets and cauliflower with a small bowl of guacamole to dip in. Add pieces of chopped fruit, in particular apples and pears because they are the toxic metal eliminators for the body. A fruit and vegie platter is a quick, nutritious meal. Make little mini salads with a dressing of olive or macadamia nut oil. A food that is very acceptable to children is a smoothie. Make it on juice, with a piece of avocado, banana, kiwi fruit or strawberries, ground almonds or macadamia nuts or add a small raw organic egg.

We have two toddlers with whom we have close contact, and their favourite breakfast is a smoothie like this, usually with the organic raw egg. These two young ladies are so advanced in ability and brain power because their little body and brain is being nourished as Nature intended.

To get lots of nutritious nuts into the diet of a small child mix fresh ground raw nuts into mashed avocado, even guacamole, grated apple or a sweet of mashed banana and other fruits. Give carrot, celery and apple juice twice daily if possible, and sneak in a small clove of garlic and a tiny piece of ginger. It may surprise you when your child freely drinks the juice.

It is okay to have a few cooked special treats and they can be made quite simply from alternate flours. Cooked sweet potato and parsnip are good replacements for potato so that there is not too much potato in the diet. Basically all children, not just autistic children, need to live on our **Primitive Diet**. Within the first week or two the change will be remarkable. Take time to read "Letters from Jasmin" in the back of this book and you'll see that a child can be 'cured' of *Autism*.

Suggested supplements
- Ester C powder - mix into a little juice twice a day
- Enysil or Floradix - a liquid multivitamin and mineral tonic especially for children

Granny's Yarns ... not!

We all have funny little sayings or beliefs passed down to us by elderly relations, friends or neighbours and we chuckle and call them 'Granny's yarns', but have you ever taken the time to really check out the validity of what they were saying? Or have you heard them talk of old remedies they always swore by till 'modern medicine' took control? We have some that turned out to be wise and true so I'll try to remember them and hand them to you to decide for yourself.

Do you remember being told to go out and pick milk thistle to rub the milk on your wart? If you did it for up to about a month your wart mysteriously disappeared. Have you had a bee sting and Mum or Grandma rubbed it with blue bag once used for whitening the washing? Sodium bicarbonate dissolved in water was something the adults drank if they had indigestion. If we were out in the bush we used young bracken fern to rub on stings and bites from insects to take away the pain. And they all work! How many more of these can you think of?

To earn pocket money to save for buying Christmas presents, I used to clean the house for an elderly neighbour. His leg had been blown off at Gallipoli during the First World War so he walked with crutches and had never married because he didn't want to be a burden on a lady. Because of this we used to help by cleaning, taking out the garbage, or running messages for him. One day he gave my sister, Dianne and me a mixture he called 'suntan lotion'. There was no such thing those days, but this was made out of peanut oil and malt vinegar. From then on we always used our 'suntan lotion' at the beach and the fact was we never burned! How I wish Mr Canty was alive today. I'd ask him how he learned about oil and vinegar as protection against the sun, and I'd dearly love to ask him what other simple remedies he could pass on.

You see, he was right. Natural cold pressed oil is protection for skin against the sun. Suntan lotion is about 90-95% mineral oil - you know - the stuff that lubricates the car, petrochemicals, highly toxic! The other 5% or so are other chemicals, the lot absorbed through the skin straight into the blood stream. It was mentioned on our national news on the radio last week that researchers in Britain say the protective affect of suntan lotion has never really been proven. Amazing how quickly authorities squashed that report and nothing more was said about the matter. The cancer industry is such a big one with billions of dollars involved, I guess it needs protecting.

History proved us correct recently. Geoff and I love reading about history, ancient and modern so we read anything that comes our way on the subject. I was reading an article about the Egyptians and it explained how the Egyptians while building their pyramids, anointed their bodies with olive oil to protect them against the fierce desert sun. This made me rather excited because in my study of the Hunzas in the Himalayas I learned that they rub apricot kernel oil into their skin for protection against the hot dry summer sun and dry icy winter. In another book I read that the Marquesans in the South Pacific rubbed coconut oil onto their bodies daily to protect them from the tropical sun. Need I say more except that none of these peoples suffered from skin cancer.

We have another theory to add to this. The 'sophisticated' western population rise each morning, shower under water filled with chlorine, fluoride, aluminium and many other chemicals, scrub our skin with strongly alkaline soaps filled with chemicals and wash our hair with even more toxic shampoo. The protective coat of natural acids and oils in our skin are washed away leaving it alkaline and unprotected. If it's the weekend we go to the beach or out to play sport smothered in suntan cream for protection. We remove our own natural acid and oil to replace it with oil that is a derivative of petrochemicals, oil that's used to lubricate our car. We're a weird mob aren't we?

The oily substance or sterol in our skin, 7-dehydrocholesterol, is required to naturally react with the sun to produce vitamin D, well known as the Sunshine Vitamin. Vitamin D's main function is to regulate all vitamin and mineral metabolism, in particular to deposit calcium and phosphorus into the bones, and is essential for keeping the nervous system and glandular system healthy. The thyroid gland needs it to help manufacture hormones to use in control of the body's metabolism. A deficiency of vitamin D leads to poor health of glands and muscles, decalcified bones and the development of such diseases as rickets (in children) and osteomalacia (in adults).

Last night I uncovered more information about sunburn, this time in relation to diet. I was reading Rebecca's naturopathy notes on vitamins and minerals looking for a particular deficiency symptom. In the vitamins folder I saw that a deficiency or malabsorption of beta-carotene in the diet (usually due to illness or disease) prevents us from being able to suntan or in their words "causes us to burn very easy". From experience Geoff and I already knew this but it's always satisfying to have it confirmed. In our early days of courting and marriage Geoff had very fair skin and couldn't go outdoors without full cover. If we went to the beach he burned sitting under the beach umbrella and as a consequence had two skin cancers removed. Once I changed our diet and we took to drinking fresh vegetable juices that contained a base of carrot juice, his skin changed, he's no longer really fair nor does he burn. Now when we go out into the paddock to work, or go to the beach, neither of us burns and I also make sure that we take our bottle of apricot kernel oil mixed with a small amount of organic apple cider vinegar (see Suntan Lotion - Miscellaneous Recipes). These days Geoff's skin has a soft, golden, healthy glow.

Carrots are one of Nature's great medicines rich in beta-carotene, a powerful antioxidant, the fighter of cancer and once converted into Vitamin A in the body, helps with night vision, bone growth, immune function, need I say more. Haven't you ever been told to eat up your carrot or you won't see in the dark? Or, rabbits eat carrots and they have good eyesight and can see in the dark.

As a child when you were sick were you given some form of oil to take from a spoon? Ours was castor oil, so disgusting, so I never admitted to being sick unless it was rather obvious and I threw up. Other parents dealt out cod liver oil to their children. The oil was to purge the illness. If you were thought to be suffering from constipation you were given a tablespoon. It was a very smart practice because it did tend to clean you out the way our food is meant to. Today we replace these medicines with dangerous, synthetic drugs and if we knew the real side effects it would scare us to death, but usually the side effects aren't disclosed unless we push the point. Have you ever heard a medical practitioner say "the benefits far out weigh the risks"? That comment always worries me. The drugs handed out to us merely cover the signs that our body is not operating correctly. It's out of balance. How about getting to the bottom of the real problem?

Here are a few other quick remedies.

For nausea drink some fresh ginger tea. Two or three slices in a cup with boiling water poured on and left to sit for about 5 minutes is a great settler of stomachs. It's also an excellent headache remedy. It will relieve you of your headache in around fifteen minutes.

Diarrhoea in children and babies can be helped by feeding grated fresh apple, a tablespoon every hour until the baby or child improves. Fresh apple juice assists in the remineralising of our bodies during and after illness. At least two apples eaten each day will help regulate body processes and remove excess cholesterol, assist in relieving constipation, relieve intestinal infections, anaemia, rheumatism, bronchial diseases, and it's been said that regularly eating apples and pears helps eliminate heavy metals from the body. That old saying "An apple a day keeps the doctor away" is correct.

Lemon juice is an invaluable medicine, an unsung hero of the past. Taken with a little boiled water to make it tepid a few minutes before breakfast, it's an excellent liver tonic. Lemon juice is a powerful antiseptic and while we think of it as a mere flavouring on sea foods today, it was used across the centuries to kill bacteria. So when you have a squeeze of lemon on your oysters or fish you're really killing 92% of the bacteria on them. It only takes a small amount of fresh lemon juice to kill the bacillus of cholera, typhoid and diphtheria. Honey, lemon juice and glycerine mixed in equal parts was one of the cough mixtures I gave out to our family on the rare occasion one of them developed a cough. How simple is that! With normal cough mixtures being 95% glycerine plus a few chemicals thrown in, I know which I'd prefer to take. The lemon has such a wide range of curative properties that once no household was without a lemon. For worms in humans the crushed seeds mixed with a small amount of honey and given over a period of about seven days will expel them. Lemon has been used in everything from medicines to beauty treatments, to stain removers (is a bleach) to moth repellants in clothing and cupboards. It's one versatile fruit.

Centuries ago cabbage was known as the medicine from heaven and the doctor of the poor. Leaves were used as poultices for leg ulcers, wounds, burns, gangrene, sprains and a long list of external problems. We drink the fresh juice added to carrot juice frequently to assist our digestion, it solves the problem of constipation and totally soothes the digestive tract. People with stomach ulcers, *Ulcerative Colitis, Crohn's Disease* and *Irritable Bowel Syndrome* will find their discomfort diminish in a day or so. At the beginning I know that it appears to cause gas in the stomach and bowel, but it's really the cabbage sweeping clean the build up of waste in the digestive tract, until it passes out of the body. With my severe intolerance to grains, they cause a bowel blockage, I find by eating some fresh cabbage and by adding cabbage to our vegetable juice, it pushes through the offending, undigested grain. Years ago it was known that freshly extracted cabbage juice fed to children before breakfast three mornings in a row, would expel worms.

Garlic is also an unsung hero. It has a long history and has been used medicinally down through the ages. The Asian peoples, particularly the Chinese, used garlic. The Egyptian pharaohs had their workmen on the pyramids fed garlic each day to protect them from epidemics and even the common people of Rome ate garlic knowing it to be a powerful tonic. My mother and grandmothers used it in many of their savoury dishes. Not only was it used for flavouring it was known to be one of the most important food medicines we possess. Even modern medical science has had to admit that it does indeed hold strong medicinal properties. We have one or two cloves of garlic in all our vegetable juices twice sometimes three times a day. Because of its remarkable bacterial, antiseptic and antifungal properties I make sure I have it every day to assist in the control of my *Candida Albicans*. The properties of garlic are so wide ranging that we should just do what our mothers and grandmothers did and have a bit each day regardless.

Parsley today we regard as a garnish or a flavouring herb for our savoury dishes. Do you eat your parsley garnish when dining out? Knowing its valuable mineral content I always eat it first. How often do you chop it and add it to your salad to increase the nutritional value of your salad? Parsley is first and foremost rich in iron followed next by calcium, beta-carotene, other vitamins, minerals and many important trace elements. Our grandmothers had many uses for parsley and it went into most savoury dishes and salads. I try to use it in salads as much as possible, too, knowing its rich vitamin and mineral content.

Drinking the tea of stinging nettle was one of the worst remedies my grandparents took, or so I thought. To me they were nasty, stinging, smelly green weeds. My grandfather used to ask us to go pick him some from a patch we knew of down an old laneway. Grandad had been diagnosed with high blood pressure so he boiled up stinging nettle and drank the tea to reduce it. Today it's still used in traditional medicine as a blood tonic, for blood pressure and more. I know it to be an invaluable herb for our biodynamic preparations, used for soil health on the farm.

Sage is important to me. I make us fresh herb teas for our breakfast each morning and it frequently contains a sage leaf or two. Apart from its ability to aid digestion, improve circulation and stimulate the nerve system to the mouth, heart and other organs of the upper body, I use it as a regulator of our hormones. It's been known for a long time that sage is an important herb to prevent the effects of menopause and menstruation irregularity. To our sage tea I often add catnip leaves which have a similar regulatory effect.

Thyme - did your grandmother have it growing at the back door as mine did? Snips of thyme went in all sorts of dishes. It flavoured stews, soups, casseroles and savoury dishes. Thyme we know is a powerful antiseptic, a nerve tonic, a stimulant for the digestive, respiratory and circulatory systems plus more. I put fresh thyme in our herbal tea for breakfast each morning and frequently add it to salads, particularly when tomatoes have been added.

These granny's yarns and practices have had an enormous influence on our everyday living and much of it we use each day. And when I think about my precious grandmothers, *I believe my grandmothers were unconsciously practising preventive medicine.*

To Live Like a Hunzakut...

Have you ever heard of Hunza?

The small principality of Hunza, now belonging to Pakistan, is hidden deep in the Himalayan Mountains amid rich glacial valleys. On the north-west boundary they have Afghanistan, north-east is China and to the south lies Pakistan. The Hunzas go back 2,300 years ago to Alexander the Great when he was conqueror and ruler of the known world. It's said that three of his soldiers deserted from his army and with their Turkish wives they fled to a hidden valley known as the Hunza Valley. These people and their descendants have farmed and lived self sufficiently since that time, hidden in their valley away from the 'civilised' world.

The reason I'm telling you about them is because, ever since I was a child I've had a passion to learn about these Hunzakuts, as they call themselves. I knew they lived to an average age of 120 years and up to 140, but I was really surprised not so long ago when I discovered they ate a basic, almost *primitive*, diet as we have the last twenty plus years. I was so excited that I decided I needed to search for more information. This came by the most amazing coincidence. I was discussing food and health with a lady on the phone one morning when I mentioned the Hunzas. She told me she just happened to have an old book, mostly pictorial, on the Hunzas, written in 1962. She would post it to me immediately. What a treasure it turned out to be! It showed the Hunzakuts living their incredible, simple life, disease-free, stress-free, crime-free; men in their nineties playing volley ball, women and children with beautiful glowing skin. I then tried to access more information on the internet and found almost nothing. My local bookshop managed to locate some old secondhand books and ordered them in for me. I just have to share with you a little of what I've learned.

Apricots are the staple food of the Hunza diet and they're eaten in some form at each meal. They contain a high quality carbohydrate and are rich in Vitamin A while another amazing attribute of the apricot is its quantity and quality of iron. Apricots were eaten fresh, the seeds were then cracked open and the kernels eaten. The kernels are an excellent and very important source of Vitamin B17. The apricots were dried on the rooftops during the heat of summer so that they could be used during the winter months of ice and snow. The kernels were also crushed for apricot kernel oil and used sparingly for cooking, and to rub into the skin for protection against Summer's sun and Winter's cold.

We're told today that you can't eat the kernels or seeds of fruit because of the cyanide content but an interesting fact is, they were used in 'the old days' as a very effective chemotherapy to cure cancer. The natural cyanide and other constituents attack the cancer cells (and cancer cells only) and this formed the natural chemotherapy till the powers that be (or perhaps a drug company?) in their wisdom decided that natural cyanide was too dangerous and deadly. The treatment was replaced with radiation, manmade drugs and chemicals with devastating side effects.

Apricot kernels in the past were used as a cheap alternative for almonds and are also the main ingredient in marzipan. When I was a teenager at school my cooking teacher asked me to help her decorate a special farewell cake with almond paste icing topped with fondant. Because almonds were so expensive due to being imported, we substituted ground almonds with ground apricot kernels. It was some years later that I learned this was called marzipan, a popular sweet in Europe, and the main reason that the attempt to ban the consumption of apricot kernels failed. Another amazing fact, in Hunza there was virtually no disease, no cancer nor any other of our western diseases, diabetes, stroke, heart disease, obesity, osteoporosis, dementia; there was no crime, no mental illness and the people cared, shared and respected each other. The communities worked together.

As well as apricots the Hunzas had a wonderful smorgasbord of fruits they grew in their region. Peaches, plums, apples, pears, quinces, mulberries, figs, cherries and grapes were all harvested and eaten along with their seeds. Fruits were the most important food consumed in the daily diet. The seeds themselves were a source of protein, vitamin C and B, and with fibre and flesh rich in vitamin A and C and you have a very impressive food. Mineral rich apples are an important medicine food. They aid digestion while their pectin content is known to expel toxins from the body. When you read of old cultures such as these and study their diet you have to wonder why our dietitians and nutritionists tell us that we should only eat 3 - 4 pieces of fruit a day, that any more is bad for us! What would *Primitive Man* have eaten? Fruit!

Vegetables were next on their list of importance. More than 70% of vegetables were eaten raw. Wood in Hunza was a sparse commodity, and since animal manure was needed for compost, they had only grass and twigs for burning. Any cooking was done for a minimum amount of time in a minimum amount of water and usually consisted of a mixture of grains and vegetables. Liquid left from cooking was used as vegetable stock. Nothing was wasted. Many kinds of vegetables were grown. Potatoes brought in by English travellers just a few centuries ago became important because they kept through the cold winter months when fresh vegetables were scarce. During summer some of the vegetables were dried so they could be added to chapattis, stews or cereal in winter. Carrots store well, as do turnips, parsnips, onions and melons. Other foods included tomatoes, capsicums/peppers (later additions, seeds from travellers passing through), beans, cucumbers and leafy greens including dandelion greens. The Hunzakuts enjoyed their corn on the cob raw, brought in fresh from their farmed terraces. Main grains were millet and some wheat. These they ground between two rocks and used immediately. Preparation method and the time it took, grain consumption would have been minimal to that of our western diet today.

Legumes, soya beans, garbanzo and lentils were grown and eaten fresh, sprouted, dried or ground. Fresh, raw soya beans are a rich protein food.

Nuts were another very important food. Walnuts were plentiful and left in their shells till they were to be eaten. Almonds were grown and are known to be the most nutritious of all the nuts, being rich in iron,

77

calcium, B vitamins, potassium and also some vitamin D. Nuts and dried fruits were carried on trips to be eaten as a meal and also formed part of their food when working out in the fields.

The only milk products consumed were mostly made from yak's milk or a very small quantity of goat's milk. Yak's milk is very rich and heavy with cream so it was made into butter and was stored away to mature. The natural enzymes and bacteria in the raw milk cause it to set into a junket ie forming a white curd leaving a liquid called whey (remember Little Miss Muffett eating her curds and whey?) Milk eaten this way has already been partially digested because of the actions of the live enzymes.

Due to the lack of space to grow fodder and the amount of feed needed to keep livestock, the Hunzas kept only a few beasts, so it was an uncommon treat to eat meat. Apart from yaks and a few goats, on rare occasions Marco Polo sheep were killed to be eaten at festival time and special celebrations. Meat wasn't served in great quantities but was cooked in a stew with vegetables for all to share. Chickens weren't allowed in Hunza because they ate grain and the Hunzakuts regarded seed more valuable than chickens.

One more important detail to mention is their water. The Hunza Valley is a glacial valley and water rushes down through rocks from the melting glaziers above, picking up minerals and trace elements as it goes. It's so rich that to see it in a drinking glass it actually appears white. This mineral rich water they drank while working in the fields and it was said to be as good as a meal. Although Hunza receives very little rainfall they were always assured of water due to the melting glaciers above.

Because of their diet and simple serene life, the Hunzas had no crime, so no need for police. They shared and cared, they knew that they had to depend on each other for survival in such a harsh countryside. They knew no illness or stress and enjoyed incredible mental and physical health and wellbeing. The men in particular still laboured in the fields up to 100 years of age. When they died it meant their time was up and they went to sleep and didn't wake. When did you last hear of someone elderly going into a peaceful sleep and simply not waking? These days there's always an illness of some kind to blame.

Women ceased to bear children in their 50's but men continued to father children into their 90's. To lose a baby was a rare occurrence and accidental death was usually the cause of death of children. Children being typical the world over, they climb, fall, break bones. In Hunza, broken bones were set by a special person in the village and usually healed in three weeks.

The reason I told you about the Hunzas in past tense is due to the phone call I had recently with a tour operator who'd been on trips into Hunza. She said that since a proper road had been pushed through the mountains, the western world had infiltrated the valley. Smoking is becoming a common practice and our western diet has sneaked in. Hence our western diseases are starting to take their toll.

Have You Heard of the Marquesans?

The Marquesa Islands are a group of islands said to be a Polynesian paradise just south of the Equator. The islands are rugged and volcanic, rising up out of the South Pacific to a height of 5000ft/2600mtrs. The valleys are of rich volcanic soil supporting an abundance of food and water.

Imagine the vision of these people to early Europeans - the men around 6ft/1.8mtrs tall, athletic, agile and strong and the women were shorter, slender and beautiful. They all had perfect dazzling white teeth, even the old people. Being islanders, they were all superb swimmers and they swam before they could walk. It was nothing for them to go for long swims each day, to another bay for an outing or around the island just for something to do. Often they took food with them and if they were hungry while swimming, they would tread water and eat. Each day, to protect them from the tropical sun they would rub coconut oil into the skin of each other, which was also a sign of affection for each other.

Breadfruit was their staple food. It was peeled, ground into a paste with stone and steamed. Bananas, fish or other foods were wrapped in breadfruit leaves and along with a pig or goat were rolled into a pit of hot stones, covered with a mat then dirt and left to slowly cook for hours. Everyone gathered to partake of the feast. The remainder of their diet was taro root, bananas, mangoes, coconuts, shellfish and fish. These fish were mostly eaten raw, caught in rock pools and eaten on the spot. Coconut was used in many ways. The immature coconut was fed to babies and children, the flesh of the mature nuts was grated and coconut cream was extracted and used with other fruits and vegetables. Bananas were the second most important food to the Marquesans and considering there were about 30 varieties that grew on the islands they were not hard to come by. One of the delicacies of these people was seafood marinated in a mixture of lime juice, coconut milk and/or sea water. They loved to eat crabs from the rock pools in the moulting season when their shells were soft. The Marquesans would come together for a feast, they would catch the crabs and pop them into their mouths whole, then chew.

These people lived in a totally natural habitat till white man came to exploit them, first trading whisky, sugar and other foreign foods for copra. Next there were the Chinese who sold sweets, canned goods and opium. Missionaries came to enforce their religion, banning the Marquesan traditions and cultural heritage. Finally French rule was the last nail to their coffin. The intruders introduced all of their infectious diseases previously unknown to these handsome people, diseases including smallpox, diphtheria, tuberculosis and syphilis, and due to the effects of their new western diet they had no resistance. By the 1920's there were only 1000 Marquesans left. Eventually after all the damage was done, the intruders left and although still under French rule, with the determination and leadership of some surviving elders who remembered the old ways and traditions, the Marquesans are on the way back.

Genetically Modified Food... What's that?

"Genetic engineering is the largest food experiment in the history of the world - and this experiment is being conducted on humans, not rats."

This statement was made by Bobby Jennings on the web site of *Holistic Politics*. His few words explain it all.

Genetic engineering is a new and scary science of which the outcome is unknown. It involves the insertion of genes of one species into another unrelated species permanently altering its genetic make up. And it gets worse...to carry out this process scientists utilise bacteria, viruses and antibiotic-resistant genes as the promoters or carriers/agents. This new genetic makeup then passes on to the offspring through heredity. In other words, this becomes the new species.

In the word of Ronnie Cummins of the American *Campaign for Food Safety* "Gene engineers all over the world are now snipping, inserting, recombining, rearranging, editing and programming genetic material. Animal genes and even human genes are randomly inserted into the chromosomes of plants, fish and animals creating heretofore unimaginable transgenic life forms."

The health implications here are insurmountable! We must remember that once the genes of plants, fish, animals and humans are altered they remain that way forever. The process can't suddenly be reversed should the scientists discover that they have made a terrible mistake.

Then we come to the use of viruses, bacteria and antibiotic resistant genes as promoters / agents. One of the main promoters used, CaMV, is a virus that genetic engineering biotechnologists argue, appears naturally in the vegetables we eat everyday. According to Dr Ma-wan Ho, a leading geneticist and biophysicist in the United Kingdom, in Nature viruses such as CaMV have a protective protein coat which prevents the virus from entering mammalian cells (that is human and other mammals) 'because its protein coat is specific to plant cells'. When it is taken from Nature and used as a promoter for gene transplanting it is 'in the form of naked viral DNA (that is, without its protein coat) and naked DNA of any sort is highly infectious'. CaMV promoter has a very similar structure to other viruses and is a close relation of *Hepatitis B* and *HIV*. The fear of using these viruses as promoters and carriers is that they may combine within a host causing new super viruses.

Could is this be where the new virus, SARS began? If my information from the internet is correct, one of the biotechnology companies stated that China has embraced the new genetically modified/engineered foods and the people show no ill affects. Where did SARS rear its ugly head? China. Canada also suffered badly from the affects of SARS. From the newspaper reports and national news on TV and radio, Canada has had GM crops forced on them for sometime. The European Union is fighting to keep genetic modified/engineered food and crops out of Europe and to date they have had no incidence of SARS. Australia has very little contaminated food yet. Our SARS cases, all three, came in from the before mentioned countries.

SARS (*Severe Acute Respiratory Syndrome*) is a new, unknown virus. It was mentioned on our national news today that the World Health Organisation has been unable to identify the virus concerned so the cause has also not been found. We are advised to be very wary and to be checked out thoroughly if we display any of the symptoms. The danger from *SARS* has not yet passed. Is this just the beginning?

Biotechnology scientists, as they like to be called, argue that genetic engineering is no different to traditional forms of breeding. In traditional breeding and Nature it is similar species that cross to produce offspring with some traits of both parents but producing a new breed. Nature also takes care here. The offspring are nearly always infertile so the species goes no further. An excellent example is a mare crossed with a donkey, the offspring becomes a mule, but the mule is infertile. When a plant, for example a flower such as a rose is crossed, a plant grown from the seed produced will not grow true to type, it will revert to the dominant parent's form. Hence the reason new varieties of plants and trees are propagated for market by striking cuttings or grafting onto other rootstock.

Gene engineering is not part of Nature. It allows scientists to plant foreign genes into animals, humans, plants ... and as Geoff always says, "For every action taken there is a reaction." What is the reaction going to be? What are these arrogant scientists, who believe they have the right to meddle with the health and well being of life on our planet, unleashing on us? Or with *SARS* are we seeing the beginning of what's to come?

I feel like I'm preaching, and I suppose I am, but we need to act now. It's time to show People Power. Take responsibility for your own life. Obtain a list of GMO foods and boycott these products. Try to buy certified organic produce for the health of yourself and your families. Avoid processed foods. According to my research, in USA it is the expectation of the biotechnology industry that 100% of food will be genetically modified in the next 5 - 10 years! Try to obtain old heirloom seeds (these biotechnology companies and their billions of dollars have already bought up the natural seed companies). Try to find a branch of *Seed Savers of the World* get some seed and grow your own in your backyards, or on your balconies. Get together with other families or neighbours and find a plot where you can all grow and share your food. We have to act now if our children are to have a tomorrow.

Foods already genetically modified/engineered in USA - soybeans, corn, potatoes, squash, canola, cotton seed oil, papaya, tomatoes, dairy products. Work is being done on fish, in particular Atlantic salmon to make them grow very large and fast for market, and then pigs. Biotechnologists are experimenting with genes from humans into pigs. They say that future organ transplants for humans could come from pigs. Does this mean that diseases from pigs will be transferred to humans as well? What if pigs are for human consumption? Does that make us cannibals?

In Australia the multinational drug companies responsible for this new technology have been waving their billions of money and pushing for the growing of commercial GM crops of canola, as well as new GM varieties of wheat. The trials of GM canola in the southern state of

Tasmania and Western Australia created such havoc that the growing of GM crops has been banned in these states.

Please go onto the world wide web and bring up 'Genetically Engineered Foods'. Check also the other countries' sites - 'Genetically Engineered Foods UK, EU, Australia, New Zealand, China, Japan' and see the controversies that are erupting.

- Genetically Engineered Foods Causing Some Concerns
- Genes from Genetically Engineered Foods Could be Detected in Brain
- Eminent Scientists Comment - here you can read what leading medical scientists are saying
- Michael Meacher Meets Scientists - this is a meeting between scientists and Michael Meacher, Minister For the Environment, United Kingdom
- Summaries of Dangers of CaMV Virus Used in Genetic Manipulation
- Hazards of Genetically Engineered Foods and Crops

Do your own research and become aware of the dangerous human experiments being forced on us. For further reading purchase a copy of *Acres* newspaper, a newspaper that will tell you the truth of what's happening. A 'must read' book, *Seeds of Deception* written by Jeffrey M.Smith, also exposes the terrible truths about genetically engineered foods, with warnings from US Food and Drug Administration scientists of new diseases, allergies and introduction of dangerous toxins into our food chain.

The sites listed below also provide information you need to know.

- **Institute for Science in Society** - www.i-sis.org
- **Physicians and Scientists for the Responsible Application of Science and Technology** - www.psrast.org
- **Australian GenEthics Network** - www.zero.com.au

I urge you, please boycott genetically modified foods, buy organic/

biodynamic foods. People power can help save our planet and leave something for our children.

Footnote : At the time of this book going to print, bees are dying in their thousands in the USA. First, authorities were blaming a mystery disease from Australia (our bees are all alive and well!) then they say they can't find a reason. On my recent visit to U.S. people involved with organic/biodynamics were freely talking about the bees feeding on GM crops as the real cause of the mass destruction of bee populations. This is the most likely reason. Monarch Butterflies feeding on the early sowings of GM canola in Canada, met a similar fate.

About Our Food

There's a lot of conflicting advice out there about food and diet and I wouldn't blame anyone for becoming very confused. I listen or read, then I ask questions and try to reason out whether what I've just heard or read makes good commonsense, and if it's simple.

Last week I was disappointed when reading an article in the children's section of my favorite magazine. There was the food pyramid of the five food groups, and listed on the bottom level, the food we supposedly require the most - grains! When I was a child grains were not that important, apart from a bit of bread, a slice or two toasted for breakfast and maybe sandwiches on a picnic, then a biscuit or a piece of cake on weekends for us was pretty special food. Our main foods were fruit and vegetables. Cooking in high school involved learning about nutrition, which included the food pyramid demonstrating the order of importance of our food groups. The food pyramid never listed grains on the bottom. I'm told that it was changed just a few years ago.

So from this grain we're encouraged to eat, we have a myriad of breads, cakes, biscuits ... and then we have pasta. But have we ever questioned what food value there really is in pasta? Unless you search out the wholemeal variety, it's mostly made from white wheat flour, sometimes with egg, but with all it's processing where are the live enzymes? How can it nourish our live bodies? Wheat is second only to dairy food for causing allergic reactions and forming mucous in our systems. The gluten is the major problem with *Coeliac Disease*, causes major problems with *Irritable Bowel Syndrome* and a major intolerance for *Candida* sufferers.

People eating a large amount of grain in their diet become very intolerant of it, and often when we eat foods of which we're intolerant makes us retain fluid. You'll hear people say that when they started to diet, they lost was an enormous amount of fluid, because they cut out breads, cakes and biscuits. I quote a personal experience here. A long time friend who was sadly overweight stayed with us some years ago. His normal diet consisted of bread, cheese and peanut butter - all unnatural, allergy causing foods. During his stay we fed him lots of salads and fruits and even conned him into vegetable juices at night and grapefruit and lemon juice for breakfast. We fed him well during the week he was with us but he lost 5kgs because we weren't feeding him those foods of which he was intolerant. He was ecstatic but went back home and resumed his usual diet!

I noticed at the top of the food pyramid in my magazine there was a gap and I'm assuming it was meant to have fats and oils in it. Medical scientists are promoting fat, especially animal fat, to be the cause of obesity. How is it that some of the old civilisations flourished on animal fats? My own grandparents lived to a good age and none were obese and they ate fat. We must have fat in our diet. From fats and natural oils (not processed vegetable oils) we get some of our essential vitamins, minerals and all important essential fatty acids. A colleague with whom I worked for a period of time decided fat was bad for her because it was being broadcast on the news, on TV, in her favourite magazines, so she cut all fat from her diet. She quickly became very gaunt and her skin seemed to age over night. We can't do without fats whether they call them good fats or bad fats.

Meat is another one of our excesses. As western countries have become more affluent, over-indulgence in meat has escalated obesity and major health problems as well. As children we ate only a small amount of meat. My dad always went to the butcher's before breakfast and brought back the next 2 days' meat. If we were having steak, it was a cheaper cut that could be sliced into a small serving for each of us and braised. We were given a lamb cutlet or half a large lamb chop each, or a couple of spoonsful of stew. Chicken was a Christmas treat. Dad killed the rooster and dressed him for Christmas dinner, and would you believe that rooster fed eight of us. Once the meat was the accompaniment to the vegetables, now we're served the meat with a spoonful of vegetables or salad as the accompaniment. Further on, I've shared some of the results of my research into two old civilisations of people, from remote parts of the world. When you read what I've learned about the Hunzas and Marquesans, their simple life and healthy diet of unprocessed and mostly raw food, you'll have to admit that the western world has lost the plot.

Think back - how many in your school class were overweight? In my class of 53 pupils there were two who were obese, the other pupils were all very normal slim to medium build, depending on their bone structure. Today, as well as our meat, dairy and grain intake we have highly refined and processed vegetable oils. As kids we only knew of castor oil, cod liver oil and olive oil. If you mentioned that you felt sick, castor oil or cod liver oil was given to purge the illness (so you bravely said nothing unless it was obvious because you threw up!) Olive oil lived in the bathroom cabinet and was used medicinally to remove cradle cap from the baby's head or drops in ears helped relieve earache, something that still works like magic.

For cooking before oils we used a little dripping - beef and lamb fat, lard from pork for special recipes, or used a bit of butter. Mum sometimes clarified the butter and we used ghee. Now we have an 'impressive' range of oils in our supermarkets and apart from cold pressed olive oils, most of them are highly refined and processed. They're stored in *clear plastic bottles* absorbing chemicals and hormones from the plastic, and going rancid in the bright lights. How nutritious! Canola oil is one of my pet hates, especially its rancid taste. Quite a number of years ago research showed that canola oil was suspected of being carcinogenic, that is, it can cause cancer, and now there can be no guarantee that it's not made from genetically modified crops either.

Let's not forget margarine here, either. What can I say about it but that it's virtually a man made synthetic food. Why do we allow ourselves to be conned by the big multinational companies who can afford to pour billions into the advertising of their products? I think the most conned of all are our doctors, nutritionists and dietitians. How have we allowed ourselves to stray so far from nature? It's time for us to ask ourselves "Does this product contain anything live to sustain good health?"

It's time for us to be responsible for ourselves rather than relying on others to do it all for us. Only we can solve our problems, and that includes our own health problems. Learn to read your body.

Remember that an allergy comes on within about 15 minutes and a food intolerance usually doesn't show up until about two days have passed. To find out what foods are reacting with you leave those that you suspect out of your diet for a week or two to allow all traces to be eliminated from your body. Reintroduce them one at a time and take particular notice over a number of days to see if there is a reaction. This should give you a true indication. I pass on a personal example here – my husband, Geoff and I ate some brown rice a couple of weeks ago. It was a cold day and I'd read a wonderfully, delicious rice recipe in a magazine…and yes we're weak at times too and eat things we know we shouldn't! Minutes after we'd eaten our rice meal both of us felt incredibly tired and felt we needed a sleep. Within a day or two my legs were heavy and it was tiring to walk up stairs and up the hill to our cabin. For me – I know my bowel wasn't working as efficiently as it should have been. A cabbage was fetched from the garden and a very nice coleslaw served up at dinner. We don't eat the same vegetables all the time, I try to vary them. We hadn't had cabbage for a few days but I went for it and made sure we had some good servings for the next 2 or 3 days, adding it to our vegetable juice as well till we returned to normal. We made a point of eating an extra apple each day for the same reason.

We noticed a long time ago that if our son, Danny ate grain as in bread or cakes, his stomach was quite noticeable. Now we've taken the time to notice, with both of us we develop a 'stomach' too. Recently I shared a lovely lunch hour with our daughter, Rebecca at a spot called *The Sushi Train*. There were lots of raw salmon and tuna, seaweed, avocado and cucumber and of course rice. Next morning back home on the farm, I dragged myself out of bed, my head felt very tight and heavy, and my legs didn't seem to want to move. Geoff that same day had attended a function in Melbourne. By Saturday he'd crashed! I asked the usual question, "What did you have to eat or drink?" He confessed to drinking two glasses of wine. Beer, wines with their preservatives and colourings (mostly sulphur - read the label on the bottle), and vinegars, anything fermented, affect the liver and especially us *Candida* sufferers. Our brave liver has the massive task of trying to detoxify all the unnatural foods, chemicals and additives with which we insult our bodies.

You'd think that since we know the consequences of our actions that we'd be wise enough to leave these things alone! The old saying I hear over and over "this little bit won't hurt" couldn't be further from the truth.

And, food for thought - it's been said that our bodies aren't biodegradable anymore, that we no longer decompose after death. Why? Because we eat so many chemicals and preservatives in our food it prevents our bodies from decaying.

About Grains and Legumes

I sometimes become frustrated when people ask me questions about our diet and way of life but in reality they want to have an argument. Last year at a literary carnival in Sydney it was very refreshing to have an in depth discussion with a fellow, Peter, as to the 'why and why not' of eating grains.

Peter said he'd spent considerable time researching natural diets and he'd been living on raw foods and without grain for more than a year. His comments were "Of course we're not meant to eat grain. We're not birds! We don't have a crop and we don't eat grit to grind up grain in our digestive system". And to be truthful I hadn't thought of it that way but immediately I knew we were on the same wavelength.

So what do we have to do to grain for us to digest it? First we grind it, we mix it with some liquid, then we cook it. It's become a foreign substance, all it's live enzymes and nutrients are dead and then we expect our digestive system to digest it. What's natural about all that?

Peter and I had a great chat about primitive man and what he would have eaten, and gorillas. Peter had been studying gorillas. He felt that if raw fruits and vegetables could satisfy and nourish these magnificent animals then why not us, after all they are supposed to be our cousins! I must say Peter looked the picture of health. He said he felt great and had enormous energy but because he carried no excess weight friends and family believed he was unwell. We constantly encounter the same attitude and comments from people around us. How quickly we accepted obesity as being the norm!

Appearing on the counter of our local pharmacy at the moment is a mat with a table of human weight to height comparisons. This is supposedly an aid for the pharmacy assistant to work out our ideal weight - are we underweight or overweight? Out of curiosity I asked one of the girls about calculating my size. She looked long and hard at me when I gave her my weight as 7st7lb/47 kilos and height as 5ft4ins/1.63mtrs. There I was positioned right down in the middle of the yellow, very under weight almost anorexic section of the table. I laughed and told her not to be concerned. I haven't had the flu for more than 20 years, the only time I have an upset is when I overindulge in a wrong food; and I have strong bones. I live and work mostly outdoors, often doing the work of a man, in sunshine, heat and cold using oil and vinegar as skin protection. I eat more than a lot of men but it's the food I eat that makes the difference. I politely told her that the conventional medical industry shouldn't generalise about these things, and who has the right to decide who is underweight.

The subject of dried legumes is another bone of contention. I've never been fond of dried legumes and pulses, and so over the years have eaten very little of them. At any time I have bothered to serve them, the whole family seemed to suffer an upset. You know the old joke? Eat baked beans and people will avoid you because of the flatulence to follow. Perhaps our bodies are saying "please don't eat dried beans!" An old naturopath over 20 years ago told us not to replace Danny and Rebecca's dairy food with soy products. They are quite difficult for the body to digest. Not that I knew anything about soy at that time, but he said consuming dried legumes causes excessive acidity in the body. It's not a natural food for us to eat.

In this category of legumes is the peanut originally from ancient Peru. The peanut causes our system to become very acidic and it also carries a type of yeast likely to cause allergic reactions. Most people are intolerant of peanuts and only the South American and African peoples are said to have evolved to be able to eat them.

Then we have the almighty multinational companies and doctors telling us, that the reason Asian women, Japanese and Chinese in particular, don't suffer from menopause is because they consume large amounts of soy products. We need to check what these wise people don't eat - dairy food, large amounts of red meat or large amounts of grain other than their ration of rice. We discovered for ourselves what the Japanese people eat on a recent visit to Japan. With our friends Hiro and Keiko we talked about diet and foods. They didn't eat dairy food and hadn't before tasted cheese. Our exciting and very different meals consisted of fish - raw, smoked and dried, lots of seaweed, some fresh tofu and vegetables and rice. We were rather amused when visiting the local *Sushi Train* for lunch one day because, as I watched the plates of food whizzing passed me I realised all the seafood was raw, but the vegetables were cooked. It was a very enlightening trip.

As mentioned in the book *Your Life in Your Hands - Understanding Breast Cancer*, Professor Jane Plant talks about her breast cancer experiences, and how the Chinese don't understand our fascination with dairy food. We westerners should be taking note. Diseases such as breast cancer (and prostate cancer for men) are almost unknown in China. Breast cancer is referred to as 'rich woman's disease', as only rich people can afford to buy dairy food and it's the rich people who develop cancer. Jane Plant's cancer resurfaced numerous times before she realised the cause.

And to the matter of these soy products in our supermarkets, how are they manufactured? To be packaged and on the supermarket shelves they have to undergo some form of processing, pasteurisation, cooking, who knows? And they just have to add nutrients, 'fortified' always worries me especially if it's calcium - often a form of powdered chalk. If it's a natural, fresh food it shouldn't need fortifying.

About the matter of soy products and menopause … I am at the age for menopause. I've not suffered any of the symptoms women complain of except once when we'd been away travelling and it had been incredibly difficult to eat our normal food. I do remember we'd eaten some breads and meat that were unnatural to us. At that time I did suffer from a couple of hot flushes that I considered weren't normal. Perhaps this means a change of diet, remove grain and legumes and eat lots more fruits and vegies and you too can be free of menopausal symptoms.

The more questions we ask about our food and the more we read our bodies, the more switched on we'll be to our own health and wellbeing. Isn't this our duty unto ourselves and to our family?

My Pantry's Contents

Due to popular request I've included a list of contents our pantry and refrigerator have stashed away in them, and as asked for, there is a shopping list. If your memory needs jogging each week photocopy the list and mark what your cupboard or refrigerator is missing. Not all these foods get purchased every week of course, so anyone who looks at all the items on the list, immediately has a stress attack and says, "I can't afford all that!" … please, stay calm and I'll tell you what I do.

Not all fruits and vegetables are in season all year round, and Nature intended for us to eat what's fresh and in season as much as possible. Different lettuces are available right through the year just as they can be grown in your garden with very little attention all year round, that is, except in very cold climates. Cabbages are always in the market along with celery, carrots, spinach/silverbeet, beetroot; radishes are fast growers and you always have them too. Apples, different varieties of pears, citrus and bananas are available through the year. Our other fruits are the seasonal delights. I know that once the summer fruits, especially my very favourites mangoes and lychees, have gone, then I can eagerly await such fruits as custard apples, kiwi fruit and mandarins.

It's a good idea to make a list each week and have a basic plan for the week's meals. When you find that you're running low in a particular food item, write it on your shopping list. With the nuts and seeds, when we were starting out, each week I bought about three different types in a quantity that would supply us up to a month. I have a number of large jars I store them in, in a dark cupboard, and when I find I'm getting low in a certain nut or seed, I replace it on shopping day. It's good to have a reasonably quick turnover in nuts so they remain fresh and don't have a chance to go rancid. I attempt to keep an amount of dried fruits as well, but there are large two-legged rodents in our house that quietly raid supplies and slink away trying to appear innocent, so mostly they are purchased weekly. The organic dried fig, heavenly dried apricot, nectarine, date and sultana jars are very difficult to keep full.

Dried herbs and spices, I'm sure you will already have in your kitchen pantry. Fresh herbs need to be purchased each week as you require them, although there is a simple solution to the fresh herbs situation. They are very easy grow and are extremely tough. Grow some either in pots if you are a high rise apartment dweller, or plant them into your flower or vegetable garden. Bees love the flowers on herbs and it brings them in to pollinate other plants. Herbs are beneficial to your vegetables and flowers, repelling many of the bad insects and bugs.

Nuts and seeds should be purchased from a store that has a good turn over in stock so there is a fair guarantee they are fresh and not rancid. If you purchase grains, much the same applies. Always strive for organic/biodynamic produce and products so you know the food you eat isn't genetically engineered, smothered in chemicals and grown with artificial fertilisers, *and* they have been grown according to Mother Nature's rules which means they actually contain the nutrients they are meant to have.

Eggs are another problem. Here in Australia some months ago I listened with disbelief to one of our nutritionist celebrities stating that our commercial poultry hasn't been fed growth hormones since the early 1950s, that hormones were banned. What she neglected to mention was, years ago it was found that by feeding chickens antibiotics they grew much faster. She stated rather strongly that it was incorrect that these birds and their eggs were detrimental to our health, and all eggs were equal. Even to buy day old chickens now, for those wanting to start raising hens, the chickens have been fed antibiotics mixed in their food and they've been vaccinated against various diseases. Other members of my family chuckled at our elderly dad because he declared his hens to be genetically modified. Our dad was a smart old man. While they chuckled at him he was closer to the truth than they realised. He was waiting for one of his hens to go broody so she would sit on some eggs and hatch chickens, but none would go broody. His hens had been purchased as pullets from a company in Sydney, and what Dad didn't realise, the pullets were the variety that had been bred and interbred (mostly inbred) to be used as battery hens, that is, to live with many thousands of other hens in unhealthy cages, in sheds. They have their beaks chopped to stop pecking and are fed all day and all night on grain and antibiotics. Their instinct to go broody has been bred out of them. Did you know that when you eat ordinary chicken from the supermarket it's taken just six weeks from day one to being in the supermarket refrigerator?

Fish and prawns purchased from the supermarket are also of concern. I was told by a fellow who once worked on a prawn trawler, that the moment prawns are caught, they're treated to keep them fresh until they get them to land and market. I believe fish is treated in some way also. I have a little more delving to do on this one.

Shopping List

Vegetables

Carrots
Cabbage - red or green
Celery
Spinach or silverbeet
Broccoli
Lettuces
Rocket/arugula, mizuna, endive
Beetroot
Fresh mixed sprouts
Cucumber
Radishes
Capsicum/red peppers
Garlic
Shallots, spring onions
Fennel
Zucchini
Peas
Beans (fresh)
Asparagus
Potatoes (non-genetically modified!)
Eggplant/aubergine
Parsnip
Pumpkin
Corn
Turnip, swedes (rutabaga)
Brussel sprouts
Onions - brown, white, red

Fruit

Apples
Pears
Bananas
Avocados
Tomatoes
Paw paw/papaya
Kiwi fruit
Mangoes
Pineapple
Oranges, mandarins
Lemons, limes
Grapefruit
Plums
Apricots
Peaches, nectarines
Cherries, blueberries
Strawberries, raspberries etc
Grapes
Custard apples
Figs
Passionfruit

Melons

Water melon
Rock melon/cantaloupe
Honey dew melon

Herbs

Parsley - curly or Italian
Coriander/cilantro
Thyme
Mint
Rosemary
Sage
Lemon balm
Chives
Basil
Catnip
Lemon verbena
Tarragon
Dried mixed herbs
Paprika
Fennel
Dill
Caraway seed

Spices

Cumin - ground or whole
Cardamom - ground/seeds or pods
Ginger - fresh or powdered
Cinnamon - ground and sticks
Nutmeg - ground/whole grated
Mixed spice
Turmeric - fresh / powdered
Mustard - ground / seed
Pepper - corns / ground
Chilli - powder/dried/fresh

Cayenne
Mace - pieces / powder
Fenugreek - ground
Allspice/pimento - ground/whole
Vanilla - essence / bean

Grains and Flours

Brown rice
Brown rice flour
Polenta, cornmeal/maizemeal
Cornflour (from corn not wheat!)
Arrowroot
Potato flour
Tapioca flour
Quinoa – grain/flour
Amaranth - grain/flour
Coconut flour

Dried Fruits

Sultanas
Currants
Raisins
Dates
Dried figs
Prunes
Apple
Pear
Apricots
Pineapple
Peaches, nectarine

Mangoes
Dried tomatoes - plain or in oil
Ginger (glaze in syrup) as a treat

Raw Nuts and Seeds

Almonds / almond meal
Macadamia nuts
Pine nuts
Pecans
Cashews - whole, pieces (cheaper)
Hazelnuts
Brazil nuts
Nut butters (or make your own)
Coconut - fresh or dried
Sunflower – kernels/seeds
Pepitas/pumpkin seeds
Walnuts

Miscellaneous
Cold pressed olive oil
Cold pressed macadamia nut oil
Cold pressed apricot kernel oil
Cold pressed sunflower oil
Cold pressed safflower oil
Eggs – organic!
Fish/other seafood not farmed
Anchovies (watch the oil for GM)
Organic apple cider vinegar
Herbamare herbal salt
Organic/Celtic sea salt
Olives (no vinegar)

Capers
Rice or corn cakes or crackers
Organic corn chips
Organic apple or pear juice
Organic honey (if allowed as a treat)
Organic maple syrup (if allowed)
Apple or pear juice concentrate
Coconut cream and milk
Baking powder (gluten free,
   aluminium free)
Bicarbonate of soda
Cream of tartar

Cleaning Aids

Eucalyptus oil
Orange oil
Bicarbonate of soda (bath, hand basin etc)
White vinegar (good rinse aid dishwasher)
Pure soap
Newspaper and water to wash windows

I know that when you look at this list you're going to say, "I can't afford to eat like this". Geoff and I have a peculiar sport. It's watching people going through the supermarket checkouts while waiting our turn. These people have trolleys full of processed foods, frozen foods such as pizzas, TV dinners, processed meats, sweets, chips, chocolate, cakes, coke and other equally harmful drinks. We look at the people and see how ill they look; after a while you become expert at detecting the signs. Most don't even realise they're ill, they just accept the way they feel as being normal. We then see the cost of their trolley full of artificial foods and we know that we can't afford to live like they do. Our budget is way below that of other people because we buy only fresh fruits, vegetables and nuts. Our chocolate is an organic dried fig, or a fresh date, or best of all a big bag of fresh cherries. We don't buy meat. One afternoon while waiting to buy meat for our animals in the butcher's shop, a lady was buying two small steaks for her and her husband's dinner. It came to over $10 and I was a wee bit stunned to think that the meat was for only one meal. Even my buying of organic and biodynamic fruits, vegetables and nuts doesn't blow my budget as meat would, and atleast I know we're getting produce full of nutrients and avoiding chemicals and artificial fertilisers.

So friends, rethink your budget, and just remember that you're also saving on doctors' bills. You can't afford *not* to change your diet or habits.

Notes on Ingredients

Organic versus Conventional

We try to purchase certified organic/biodynamic produce and foods over and above all else. By purchasing only certified produce you can be guaranteed of eating foods free of harmful artificial fertilisers, chemicals, and bad farming practices. Organic farmers have a certifying body to answer to, the soils have to be built up with natural composts, rock phosphates (crushed rock, definitely not super phosphate!) and green manure crops, ensuring the essential nutrients are in the soil for uptake by the fruits and vegetables. Auditors undertake regular checks on organic producers, and should anything not comply with the national and certifying bodies' standards, they have some explaining to do. Penalties can be as severe as the immediate cancellation of their organic certification.

Folk tell us they can't afford to buy organic but we can hardly be classed as millionaires, yet we manage it, because we can't afford the medical bills. This is never considered. Also, should our health have a monetary value? Our health is priceless to us, we really only have one good shot at this life, so be like us and try to make it a healthy and happy one. There is an alternative. Have you thought of growing your own?

Eggs

To begin, it's a great source of annoyance to me when nutritionists, dietitians and doctors tack eggs into the dairy food category. Cows and chickens look nothing alike to me! Cows are mammals, have hair, four legs, an udder to suckle their babies with mother's milk; chickens are birds, have feathers, fly with wings, have two legs, lay eggs and incubate them by sitting on them to keep them warm, till 3 weeks later their babies pop out. Their digestive systems are even more dissimilar. A cow has four stomachs and is able to bring food back up later, to sit and calmly chew her cud to further digest it. A chicken eats shell grit and other grit to help it grind up grain, bugs, beetles and grubs. People are led to believe that if they're allergic to dairy food then they must be allergic to eggs.

I suspect that the real reason many people have an allergy to eggs is due to a reaction to the antibiotics fed to hens, plus chemicals in the grain they eat. If the grain isn't organic then there is a good possibility that the grain is deficient of many nutrients. Add to this the fact that the eggs are laid by poor, unhealthy 'battery hens' crammed in cages in sheds, who never see the sunshine, breathe fresh air or fossick around in a lovely grassy paddock, looking for nutritious bugs, worms, beetles and insects. The saying that 'we are what we eat' applies to all creatures, not just us. Eat certified organic, free-range eggs and you'll be sure you're getting the real thing. Then see if you're still allergic or intolerant.

Butter/Ghee

Butter being a dairy food, very little or none should be eaten, *not* because it's a fat. Although it's made from the fat of the milk, it does still contain some milk solids. Should you wish to use some in the cooking you can clarify it so that you're left with ghee. Heat the butter gently on low heat in a saucepan for a couple of minutes until melted, then set aside to cool. The fat separates from the milk solids and sets on top leaving the milk solids on the bottom. Skim off the fat known as ghee and leave the more harmful milk solids behind. You then have pure fat. It's your decision if you want to use a little as a treat or in cooking. Remember it will have no real nutritious benefit.

Honey/Maple Syrup and a Replacement

First be aware that if it's not organic honey that you've purchased there is a great possibility that the bees have been fed antibiotics, supposedly to keep certain diseases at bay. To further insult one of Mother Nature's pure medicinal foods, the honey may contain liquid glucose to 'make it go further'. For what other good reason would a beekeeper have to ruin honey!

I know *Candida* sufferers shouldn't have honey or maple syrup, I'm one of them. In many recipes it's not necessary, particularly where fruit or dried fruits are concerned. For those wanting the sweetness but not the sugar try 2 to 4 dates soaked for a few hours in fresh orange or apple juice, or filtered water, it depends on how much you require in your recipe. To replace half a cup of honey I would place 4 to 5 dates in a half cup measure and fill with the juice or water. Once the dates have softened, puree them and add the mixture to your recipe…just a word of warning though, if you taste the dates and juice mixture you're likely to eat them before they make it to your recipe.

Oranges/Mandarins
Oranges contain volatile oils that can cause cystitis like symptoms in women, in particular if they have *Candida*. Mandarins will also, but to a lesser degree. These days I am more in control of my *Candida* and am lucky to be able to tolerate oranges and mandarins with no ill affects.

Peaches/Nectarines/Apricots and Pineapple
Some people with allergies and intolerances will find these fruits have a reaction similar to oranges and mandarins. I was one of these people once also. I now eat them all.

Fresh coconut Water
Fresh coconut water drained from a coconut is a highly nutritious liquid to be consumed fresh. Drink as it is or by add to smoothies and drinks.

Coconut cream
In spite of popular belief, fresh coconuts are highly nutritious and fresh coconut milk or cream can be made if you have a Green Power juicer or similar large juicer. For those who aren't fortunate enough to have one, fresh coconut milk can be made by removing the copra (white flesh) and grating it, then adding it to the coconut water from inside the coconut, or filtered water, and squeezed through a clean muslin cloth. If you need to use tinned/canned coconut cream always read the tin to make sure it has no additives.

Salt
I use unprocessed sea salt or celtic salt and I worry little about its supposed affects. We need a little salt in our diet and these salts still contain sea minerals, because they haven't been processed and refined. I sometimes use Herbamare herbal salt, which also has other ingredients beneficial

to our bodies - dried celery leaves, parsley, marjoram, rosemary, thyme, kelp etc. Never use salt fortified with iodine!

Pepper
Pepper is optional because it can be an irritant to the kidneys. A little sometimes is okay.

Guar Gum and Agar Agar
Both these gelling agents can act as mild laxatives, and although they are plant and seaweed based they could be detrimental to your health if used in a large quantity.

Alcohol in recipes
In one or two recipes you will see a little alcohol. We rarely have alcoholic beverages due to their toxic effect on the liver. Also because it's fermented and full of sugar, alcohol feeds the *Candida* yeast in the digestive system. To add a small amount in recipes for flavour, first heat it gently so that the actual alcohol evaporates. Something to watch out for too, is that wine contains the preservative sulphur, mostly numbered 220 unless label states otherwise.

Anchovies
Many Asian recipes have fish or oyster sauce added to them for flavour. Well...most fish and oyster sauces contain unhealthy additives such as MSG (monosodium glutamate). Once when I wanted to make one of these recipes, I gave considerable thought to what I could replace the fish sauce with. Then it came to me. An anchovy would give the flavour without the harmful chemicals. So, if you have a recipe that needs fish sauce or oyster sauce, mash up an anchovy or two and add to your dish. (You can always mash a fresh oyster or two if available).

Vinegar
We don't use vinegar due to the fact it's fermented and has a similar affect to alcohol. White vinegar should only be used as a cleaning agent. It's harsh and astringent. The only vinegar we do have in our pantry is organic apple cider vinegar that has been naturally fermented. I mostly use a little for our suntan lotion.

Pasta and Noodles

We have pasta as a special treat, when visitors come, but it's always gluten-free made from rice or a mixture of rice and corn. In place of pasta I occasionally serve rice noodles.

Freezing

We rarely freeze foods. Our daughter, Rebecca said vaguely to me one day that freezing explodes the cell structure of our food, but she didn't elaborate. A couple of facts I do know, sometimes fresh foods can be frozen for two weeks to kill certain bacteria, viruses or parasites, and another fact of interest, while over visiting our special friend, Maija in Finland, we went hiking through the forest. It was early Spring and the thaw was setting in. In places there were still patches of ice and under the ice were wild berries still totally preserved, not frozen, fresh as though they had just ripened. Our freezers don't preserve food like this. We were able to try so many different berries! This is a matter for me to investigate more closely in the future. Otherwise, be like us, eat fresh food in season the way Nature intended. Eat frozen food on a rare occasion.

FOR BABY

First Foods

Mother's milk...mother's milk...mother's milk
What more can I say! The most natural food invented for our human babies. Not cow's milk with its high level of calcium and protein, needed to nourish calves and their big, heavy, fast growing bones and bodies. Not goat's milk, meant for feeding gambolling kids; that is, unless Mum has problems feeding but it must be raw. Although it's the closest to human milk it has a slightly higher amount of protein than human milk. Baby kids have different needs to human babies so to feed your baby it needs to be diluted half goat's milk to half filtered water. Also, *definitely* never feed soy milk because a baby's digestion is not developed enough to process soy milk, a man made product from dried legumes. I was told by an old naturopath more than 20 years ago that dried legumes, as in soy milk, are difficult for us to digest and cause our bodies to become very acidic. If Mum is unable to feed her baby, strained raw almond milk diluted with strained fresh carrot juice will be a nourishing replacement.

Here is a small point of interest for you. Looking back to native civilisations for guidance, the native mothers of the group of islands known as The Marquesas supplemented and fed their babies the soft jelly-like contents of immature coconuts. These immature coconuts contained all the nutrients a baby required for growth and development should Nature somehow have failed them.

Introduction of other Liquids
Between one to two months of age other liquids can be introduced. Once it was strained, fresh orange juice which more often than not caused a scalded bottom. Then came the quick, easy commercial baby fruit juices - *don't* influence a baby with over sweet, processed commercial baby juices that are totally devoid of any nutritional value. An excellent alternative is fresh, raw carrot juice diluted in a ratio of one part carrot juice to three parts filtered water, a teaspoonful to begin with and slowly increasing to ½ cup. Fresh apple juice can be used in the same way. This is usually given as the afternoon snack following the afternoon sleep.

First Solids
- given when the baby is no longer satisfied with just liquids, about 4 - 6 months
Mashed ripe banana
Fresh grated or pureed apple
Fresh pureed pear
Mashed avocado
Mashed paw paw/papaya
Mashed mango
Mashed strawberries

Only one fruit at a time should be introduced and fed to the baby for a couple of weeks, beginning with bananas and only a teaspoonful till the baby has acquired the taste. By adding fresh, raw fruits you're supplying extra nourishment to aid in the development of the baby's brain and other related systems, as well as developing taste. As baby's taste develops, smoothies are a great simple and nourishing meal, especially if they have the milk from a fresh coconut or a raw organic egg. These can be given for breakfast or at any feed time. (See smoothie recipes) *Fresh, raw organic fruits are essential.* These will be free of toxic chemicals and artificial fertilisers, and be rich in all the necessary vitamins and minerals that will be in the fruit.

8 to 12 months and onwards
As well as continuing with essential mother's milk, small amounts of other salad vegetables can be introduced. Puree some salad greens and mix with mashed avocado. Not only are avocados rich in proteins, vitamins and minerals, but they are a fantastic base for soft foods. Stir in some fresh carrot juice, add a little pureed tomato, or add some grated apple or pear. By 12 months the baby can be having fresh raw pureed or finely chopped broccoli, fresh beans, celery, grated fresh carrot. It's at the early age of 6 to 12 months that a baby develops his/her taste for food. If fed bland, commercial baby food products, apart from eating dead food, a baby doesn't acquire a taste for good wholesome, flavoursome food, nor does he/she adjust to chewing anything solid or lumpy. Below are some recipes to help.

Baby's Breakfast

If you choose to feed your baby cereal when the time is right to give some form of solid food at the morning feed time, beware of the types of grain and ways of preparing them. *Never* buy packaged baby food. I attempted to feed Rebecca some once and she refused to eat it so I tried it myself. I swear the cardboard box it was in would have tasted better. I changed to mixing a little finely ground oats with milk at the time, but made rolled oat porridge on fruit juice later. Following are some recipes I've come across that you might wish to try.

Amaranth Cereal

1 tablespoon amaranth finely ground (found in health food stores)
3 tablespoons fresh apple juice
1 apple grated - alternatively mashed banana, pear, paw paw/papaya, a little peach etc

Bring the amaranth and apple juice to the boil, stirring continuously. Boil a minute or two then remove from the heat and allow to cool. Mix in the fresh grated apple or fruit and feed to your baby.

- Finely chopped organic oats can be cooked, also with fruit juice and add grated or mashed fruits. Prunes are a great addition too.

Rice Cereal

1 tablespoon finely ground brown rice
3 tablespoons fresh apple juice
¼ pear mashed, grated or pureed
Ground almonds

In a small saucepan, boil the ground rice with the apple juice till rice is cooked. Cool. Add the pear and stir. If a little too moist, stir in some ground almonds.

Quinoa Cereal

1 tablespoon quinoa
3 tablespoons fresh juice to soak cereal
Mashed banana or other fruit mashed or pureed
Almond meal/ground almonds or almond milk

**Soak the quinoa overnight in the apple juice. Next morning stir
in the mashed banana or fruit and adjust consistency with ground
almonds or almond milk.**

* Alternately boil the quinoa and juice till cooked. Allow to cool
  then stir in the fruit.

Soft boiled egg (in the old days called a coddled egg), can be given as
a breakfast food. Serve a little grated fruit followed by a soft boiled
egg. My mother always fed the baby coddled egg, an egg cooked in
its shell for a brief minute. The egg will only be partially set.

Fruit and Ground Nuts Breakfast

¼ apple finely grated
¼ banana mashed
½ tablespoon ground almonds

**Mix all together well. If the puree is a little stiff dilute with a
squeeze of orange juice or apple juice.**

* In place of ground almonds use ground macadamia nuts.

Baby Salads

Carrot and Sprout Salad

¼ avocado roughly chopped
1 tablespoon grated carrot
1 tablespoon alfalfa sprouts
1 small piece of green lettuce leaf
A few parsley leaves
A little fresh carrot juice or apple juice

Puree the ingredients till reasonably smooth and feed to Baby. Any left I'm sure other members of the family will be quick to devour. Any of the greens, broccoli, beans, lettuces etc could be added to this mixture.

Potato and Raw Vegetable Salad

1 tablespoon warm mashed potato or sweet potato
Fresh carrot juice
Pureed raw vegetables
Grated carrot

Combine all the ingredients and feed to Baby.

Tomato and Carrot Salad

¼ avocado mashed
Pureed tomato
Grated carrot

Mix tomato puree with avocado to make it a smooth consistency, then add grated carrot or for smaller babies puree the carrot as well.

Sweet Baby Salad

¼ avocado mashed
½ banana chopped or other fresh fruits mashed or chopped finely
Juice half an orange or a little fresh apple juice
1 teaspoon almond meal or macadamia nut meal

Mix together the mashed banana and avocado, then mix in juice and nut meal. Feed it to Baby and he/she will love it.

• Add 2-3 chopped prunes for variety.

Don't forget to give your baby pieces of fruit that they can pick up and eat for themselves once they are 12 to 14 months of age and have teeth with which to chew - under strict supervision of course. I used to place our two in the high chair where they could sit, all very civilised and important. I knew then that they wouldn't be toddling around with food in their hand or mouth in a dangerous manner, or scrubbing the floor or furniture with it - all part of learning discipline and manners.

By the time your toddler has reached 18 months to 2 years he/she should be able to eat very finely chopped food that the rest of the family is eating, sitting at the table in a high chair taking his/her place in the family. I always made sure that we ate breakfast and dinner together, and shared conversation of the day's activities.

There is nothing wrong with breastfeeding babies up to 2 years of age or more, just as Nature intended. If we consider peoples of the supposed 'third world countries' who haven't lost most of their mothering instincts, as we seem to have, they breastfeed their babies up to 3 years of age. Why are we made to feel backward or bad if we decide to provide for our babies the way we were meant to? That also being the case if we decide to take on the proper role that is ours by Nature – to stay home and raise our own babies. How mothers can leave their babies at day care establishments I'm not sure. Although we were a low income family I made sure that I put all my time and effort into fulfilling my duties as a mother. I loved every minute of it and I don't remember ever regretting being there, instead I remember the fun, all the endearing little habits Rebecca and Danny had and the funny things they did. Now it seems that money and the perceived need for possessions, most quite unnecessary, rates higher than the joy of raising our children. This is a full time job alone so please don't feel guilty should you choose to follow this path.

Some time ago I asked our daughter Rebecca, if she ever considered herself a deprived child because she and Danny never had the latest fads and fashions in toys, computers and games. She admitted that she never noticed they'd missed out on anything. They had wooden bats, tennis balls, shuttlecock and bats, jigsaw puzzles, wooden building blocks and an old mechano set. Then of course they had lots of Little Golden Books we used to read. We said or sang nursery rhymes and poems. We had such fun.

Another problem we face today raising our babies is the guilt heaped upon us if we dare to discipline our children. From day one babies work out their mother and father and how far they can push them. Babies cry for different reasons not just to get a feed, as is the popular belief today, and if Mum doesn't learn to interpret the baby's cries then the baby very quickly knows that if he/she bellows Mum comes running. I'm very thankful that I had great lessons taught me by my mother and grandmother. They both always said, "stick to a routine, babies love routine". Babies are born into a family, family life doesn't revolve around the baby, the baby doesn't control the family. And how right they were.

I kept to a family rhythm. I fed our baby at 5.00am when Geoff had time to enjoy the moment, then we were up in time for breakfast and Geoff to go to work. At 8 - 8.30am my baby was happy to kick and wait till it was time for a bath and next feed. Following the feed I pushed he/she outdoors in the pram to have a kick in the sunshine with his/her nappy off. A little whinge would tell me my baby was tired and I tucked him/her up for the morning sleep. Lunchtime feed was 1.00pm and my baby was always awake for it and ready to go. A change and down she/he went for the afternoon nap. Around 3 - 4 o'clock my baby was always awake again for what my grandmother called 'mothering time'. The baby was fed diluted fresh juice then it was Mum's time out to sit back, relax and enjoy playing with her baby and children.

We used to play and sing and rock in time to music. I have to admit that it happened at each nappy change as well with me. I couldn't help it, I always sang nursery rhymes and lullabies and chattered. Singing and saying nursery rhymes stimulates the baby's senses and increases awareness and alertness to his or her surroundings, as well as being fun. By 5.00pm Baby was ready for another feed then to be tucked up till 9.00pm feed. At 9.00pm Dad was around to play and help. I wet a face cloth with lovely warm water and wiped the baby's face and hands then the tail end while the nappy was being changed. This 'top and tail' freshened them up and they were slipped into their nightdress. After a feed it was into bed for the night.

Because I worked to a routine both our babies started to sleep through the middle of the night feed by the age of 4 to 5 weeks. I realised what I was doing with Rebecca, our first born. When she made a noise or movements, I would jump up and feed her. Then one night was so cold and I was weary, still recovering from the after effects of a Caesarian birth, when she started to wriggle and grunt around the 1.00am feed time, I reached over, poked her dummy in, rocked the cradle and I fell back asleep. Her cries awakened me, and when I sat up to pick her up I found it was 5 o'clock in the morning. From then on I didn't need to feed her in the night. I had actually been waking her up to feed her. This is how babies develop bad nighttime sleeping habits.

I had other good teachers at the beginning as well, right from Nature. First, my mare had a foal. At set times during the day the foal had a feed. If it wasn't feed time there was no way my mare would allow him to suckle. At set times Rocky, the foal had a sleep, at first in the morning and the afternoon. As he grew older he had only an afternoon sleep. I loved watching the fat little pink piglets up the hill in the pigsty. Mother sow always pushed her piglets away and wouldn't let her milk down if it wasn't time to feed, but the moment it was time she made all the right noises a mother pig should, and called them to her. She'd flop down and the piglets would tumble over each other to get to their teat.

Due to present day political correctness we're being stopped from disciplining our children, by giving a smack for things they do wrong. In nature programs on television have you watched lion cubs tumbling around and over their mum? If they overstep the mark with her, she gives them a nip. Vixens do the same with their fox cubs, cats do with their kittens and dogs do with their puppies. Discipline is part of an animal's survival. We're animals too remember, and our children need to be taught to respect and care for others to survive in our society.

Just like Rocky, the foal our children had afternoon sleeps right till they were 4 years old. Even if they didn't sleep they went to bed and had a rest. I frequently hear mothers say they can't get their children to bed, first in the afternoon, then at night. Who's the boss in the household? Our children were usually calm but if they didn't have their afternoon sleep they became overtired and unbearable by dinnertime. Even though they had an afternoon sleep they were down in bed by 7.30, we read books for a few minutes then without a word they went to sleep. They need to know that Mother's and Father's word is law, and mutual respect and love develops. It also adds to their feeling of security because they know their mum and dad are there for them. Children are very quick to pick up on their parents' insecurities. As they grew older we gradually allowed Rebecca and Danny to make more decisions for themselves but with our guidance where necessary. Eventually they reached a stage as young teenagers when we only had to say, "is that wise?" or "why do you want to do that?" and they reasoned things out for themselves.

And about the smacks, when they were first mobile around the floor (ours rolled around before crawling), if they touched something they shouldn't we just gave their hand a gentle smack and said, "No, don't touch". By the time they were walking they knew what they could touch and what to leave alone. I never placed precious things up out of reach and I never fastened cupboards with gadgets. When we went to other homes or out shopping it was a pleasure and fun to have them with us, and we always took them. If anything took their fancy a polite and gentle "no don't touch" was all we needed to say.

So, along the way through life, if you are ever in doubt about how to manage things, just ask yourself, how would Nature take care of it? Whether it be raising babies, eating or living, it will be relevant.

Plan a Menu

Breakfast - A Simple Affair

Fresh squeezed juices
Grapefruit with boiling filtered water to make it tepid. Grapefruit juice aids in digestion and actually helps us assimilate more of the food we eat, lemon is excellent as a liver detoxifier, for cleansing the lymphatic system and eliminating the wastes from our body. An alternative to grapefruit juice, cut grapefruit into wedges and eat before your other fruits. A glass of fresh vegetable juice is also highly beneficial.

Bowl of fresh fruit salad, fruit platter or compote
in total 2 - 3 pieces of fruit per person
Sprinkle with fresh raw nuts or serve on a platter (optional)
The list of fruits is endless.

Paw paw/papaya	Pears	Bananas	Apples
Apricots	Peaches	Grapes	Berries
Figs	Cherries	Mangoes	Kiwi fruit
Pineapples	Plums		

Eggs
1 or 2, boiled in shell - bring water to the boil in a saucepan, turn off heat and add eggs to the water for one to three minutes and they should be cooked; poached and placed on toasted rice bread, rice cake or slice of damper, or for special treat on a Sunday morning, serve Eggs Benedict with smoked salmon on a toasted slice of rice bread or damper. See Breakfast recipes.

Toasted rice cakes, damper or corn cakes (optional)
lightly buttered or spread with ghee, replace with avocado and/or spreads (see jam and spread recipes in Miscellaneous).

Herbal tea
Any mixture of herbs is fine. Below is a list of combinations -
• Lemon grass, lemon balm, lemon verbena, catnip

- Thyme, sage, rosemary, fresh sliced ginger (one of our breakfast combinations)
- Ginger and slice of lemon or lime
- Lemon grass
- Peppermint / spearmint
- Chamomile
- Other herbs include :- Red clover, hops, nettle, calendula, marshmallow, pineapple sage etc (See Beverages)

As well as making a refreshing cuppa to have at mealtimes and breaks, these are all medicinal herbs and will assist with many ailments. A couple of the very important ones are sage and catnip, a little of which we have each day. It helps women and their menopausal problems, and men stay free of prostate problems.

Between Meal Snacks

If you need a snack between meals, it's best to keep it simple. Dried fruits, raw nuts and fruit will keep your blood sugar at the right level and your brain functioning alertly. Dried fruits and nuts being raw complex foods take longer to digest so their energy is slowly released sustaining you for a longer period of time. This can't be said for all your biscuits and chocolates, you experience a "sugar hit" then crash afterward. Below is a list of goodies to take to work or play.

Any fruits from bananas to apples, pears, cherries, grapes, peaches, apricots, plums etc. Naturally dried fruits eg. apples, pears, apricots, sultanas, raisins, currants, figs, pineapple, mango, paw paw/papaya (be careful that it is not dried using sugar and/or sulphur) and add to it a mixture of nuts and seeds eg. raw almonds, pecans, pine nuts, brazil nuts, hazelnuts, raw cashews, pumpkin seeds / pepitas, sunflower seeds ….

Melons
Now would be the time to eat a good wedge of melon as melons are very quick and simple to digest, and should be eaten as a meal alone. Eat lots of watermelon, rock melon/cantaloupe, honeydew melon etc.

Melons contain over 90% of natural mineral water with an exceptional balance of minerals and some vitamins.

Candida sufferers need to be aware that rockmelons/cantaloupes have a type of yeast on their skin and by eating them you may have a reaction to them. I personally haven't had a reaction to them at all.

Lunchtime

This is the *hour* you should make sure you relax, take your time and eat a salad from the salad section, add nuts and seeds and/or especially eat fruit. Fruits, dried fruits and nuts are a very good combination to keep you bright and alert and satisfied for the afternoon. We don't eat cooked foods at lunchtime but I know that some people feel deprived if they haven't had something substantial.

The reason we feel drowsy following sandwiches or other heavy carbohydrate for lunch is that it puts a strain on our digestive systems, to eat like this at this time. Our body needs the very natural fruit sugar to boost our blood sugar level. By lunchtime it's beginning to drop. The water, natural sugar and fibre of the fruit, and dried fruit along with nuts put less strain on our digestion, and will sustain us through to afternoon tea.

- Pack a salad in a lunchbox. Add some fish. Dressings can always be made and in the refrigerator ready to use. They will keep for 2 - 3 days.
- Cook extra zucchini or corn fritters the night before and take cold for lunch or afternoon tea. Do be aware, due to the mixture of flours in the fritters, although only a small amount, they can make you sluggish.
- Fill a little box with a mixture of dried fruits and nuts.
- Take vegetable straws and florets and aioli in which to dip. Alternatively, take guacamole to dip the vegetable straws in.
- Dips and corn chips as well as salad
- Take some herbs in a little bag or box so that you can have a refreshing cup of herbal tea at any time. Just tear some pieces of herbs, throw into cup and pour on boiling water, allow to sit for 4 - 5 minutes then drink. Herbs sink to the bottom when the tea is ready.

Dinner

This meal should be predominantly raw. We should never go to sleep on a stomach full of cooked food that it's trying to digest. The food ferments in the stomach and can lead to many disorders and diseases. The reason people rise in the morning and say they can't eat breakfast because they're not hungry, last night's dinner is still trying to digest.

Choose any salads, main meals and raw sweets to make a complete and exciting meal. The choices are endless and only limited by your imagination.

Raw Vegetable Juices

The most pure and rich of liquids you can drink, raw vegetable juices are full of vital vitamins and minerals that we miss out on in our denatured foods we consume daily. These juices are all known for their own special properties and can be combined to form Nature's own medicine. Below is a brief list of some of these juices. For more information it would be of a great advantage to obtain a copy of my first 'food bible' and book of commonsense, *Raw Vegetable Juices*, now known as *Fresh Vegetable and Fruit Juices* written by Dr NW Walker, D.Sc. In his book Dr Walker explains the combinations and quantities of juices to drink to assist with various illnesses.

- *Carrot Juice* - one of the best of Nature's Medicines in preventing colds and viruses, germs and infection. Aids in the fight against cancer and disease by building up the immune system. Very important for the eyesight and skin. It builds up serotonin to protect our skin against sunburn and skin cancer. Most vegetable juice combinations have carrot as a base.
- *Beetroot Juice* - nourishes the brain and nervous system and is an excellent liver tonic. This excellent source of manganese is also essential for development of blood and bone. Beetroot is of great value to women with menstruation and menopausal problems.
- *Cabbage* - is a cleanser of the body, expelling waste matter, working as a liver tonic and acting as a broom sweeping the bowel clean.

- **Celery** - this contains the natural salts required by our body for the formation of cells. The minerals in celery assist in the cleansing of the bloodstream and elimination of toxic substances that deposit themselves in various parts of the body, causing health problems.
- **Garlic** - a powerful antifungal and natural antibiotic. It contains a large amount of natural sulphur, which helps in the elimination of mucous and toxins from the lymphatic system and entire body. It boosts the immune system and aids in the prevention of infection. This is an important anti-*Candida* food.
- **Ginger** - another powerful antifungal. It settles upset stomachs, so is essential for those who suffer from morning sickness or motion sickness, is excellent for good circulation, a warming food.
- **Silverbeet / spinach** - a great nerve tonic, a blood building vegetable due to large amounts of iron, manganese and copper.

Any vegetable can go into the juice. If you at first find raw vegetable juice unpalatable add an apple which also contains important minerals. Our children at a very young age drank vegetable juices. We explained to them that it was their natural medicine and they never argued. We rarely if ever had a sick child.

I know that I'm repeating myself, but to eat raw foods is as Nature intended, and as *primitive man* did, gathering fruits and berries from the bushes and trees, using a stick to dig up tubers from the ground and picking nuts that were hanging around in their own little packaging. I wonder how often he was lucky and cunning enough to catch an animal or fish to eat.

We've come a long way since then, now our food is gathered for us. It's grown in depleted soils full of artificial fertilizers, poisoned with sprays, and as I said, possibly genetically modified, and then can be stored indefinitely in cold storage or gases or irradiated. (Irradiation preserves food by hitting it with dangerous gamma rays 10,000 times the lethal dose to humans. This radiation destroys all food enzymes and vital nutrients in our food).

Recently I was told that some major supermarkets dip produce such as lettuces in a chlorine solution to kill harmful bacteria. The ulterior motive? It gives the produce a shelf life in the supermarket of up to 12 days. Then we can cremate our food by a microwave oven!

We live in scary times! And the Powers That Be tell us that it won't hurt us. I can't impress enough, try to buy organic as much as possible, produce is becoming more available now and though I keep being told that people can't afford it, I don't understand how they can afford the medical bills. How can you put a price on your health? We're very fortunate, in our area we have a wonderful store called Candelo Bulk Wholefood. There we can buy everything from fresh, organic/biodynamic fruits and vegetables in season, all kinds of nuts, dried fruits, flours, grains, seeds, herbs and spices to teas. The first visit is a real adventure. But, why not save yourself money, grow your own fruits and vegetables in season.

BREAKFAST

Fresh Apple Muesli

Grated apple, one per person
Raw nuts chopped, mixture or plain almonds, pecans, pine nuts,
brazil nuts, hazelnuts
Sunflower seeds
Some dates pitted and chopped (optional - can use sulphur-free
sultanas, currants etc)
Fresh grated coconut
Juice of fresh oranges or passion fruit

**Place apple in bowls and decorate with nuts, seeds, dates and
grated coconut. Pour over orange juice or drizzle with passion
fruit.**

- Delicious alternatives - peaches, apricots, mangoes, pears,
  bananas, finely chopped

Bowl of Prunes for Two

2 cups organic dried prunes
Fresh apple juice
Squeeze of lemon or lime juice
Fresh grated coconut

**Soak the prunes with enough apple and lemon / lime juice to
cover and leave over night. By morning they will be plump and
juicy. Serve in two bowls topped with fresh grated coconut.**

- Prunes can be replaced by your favourite fruit, dried but out of
  season to be fresh.

Berry Breakfast

3 cups berries
1 cup fresh fruit juice eg apple, orange, ruby grapefruit
1 cup mixed nuts chopped eg almonds, macadamias, cashews,
hazelnuts, pine nuts
Sprinkle of cinnamon or pinch of cloves or allspice

**Arrange two cups of the berries in individual bowls. Puree the
third cup and add fresh juice and spice. Pour the puree over the
berries in the bowls and heap chopped nuts on top.**

- To make the puree on top creamy and thick include a ripe
  banana.

Winter Fruit Compote

4 dried figs
8 prunes
4 apple rings
4 apricots
4 cups organic apple juice or orange juice
Good pinch of cardamom or ground cloves

**Combine the juice and spice. Soak the fruit overnight in the juice
and serve next morning for breakfast.**

- Replace dried fruits listed above with other dried fruits of your
  choice eg raisins, peaches, nectarines, mango

Fruit and Amaranth

½ cup coarsely ground amaranth
2¼ cups fresh apple juice
Grated rind of a lemon or lime
1 cinnamon stick
2¼ cups chopped fruits and berries
¼ cup chopped almonds or other nut

In a saucepan combine the amaranth, apple juice, lemon or lime rind and cinnamon stick, and bring to the boil stirring all the time. Take from the heat and leave to sit for about 5 - 10 minutes. Allow to cool a little, then remove the cinnamon stick and mix in fruits. Spoon into breakfast bowls, sprinkle with chopped almonds and serve.

French Toast My Style
Sunday Morning Special

4 thick slices of rice bread
4 organic free range eggs
Dash vanilla
2 cups fresh fruit or berries chopped or pureed
Cinnamon
A little organic oil for the frypan

Beat the eggs and vanilla in a flat-bottomed bowl and dip in both sides of the bread slices. Gently fry in the pan on each side till golden. Take from the pan and arrange 2 slices per person on warmed plates. Sprinkle slices with cinnamon and spoon over the fruits or puree and eat. A great Sunday morning breakfast.

Boiled or Poached Eggs with
Fay's Dukkah or Dukkan

1 - 2 organic free range eggs per person
Slices of toasted damper, rice bread, rice or corn cakes
Butter or ghee (optional)
Prepared Dukkah or Dukkan (see in Lunch recipes)

**Boil or gently poach eggs, sprinkle with dukkah or dukkan and
serve with toast.**

Eggs Benedict

4 organic free range eggs poached
4 slices smoked salmon
4 toasted slices rice bread or damper
Parsley and/or thin lemon wedges to garnish

Hollandaise Sauce
4 organic free range egg yolks
125gms/4oz butter or ghee
1½ tablespoons lemon juice
Organic sea salt
Grind fresh pepper

**Divide butter/ghee into thirds and place 1/3 in the top of a
double boiler with the egg yolks. Gently cook over hot water (not
boiling) stirring all the time until the butter/ghee melts. As you
stir in another third of butter you'll notice sauce start to thicken.
Add final third of butter and stir quickly till melted. Remove
from the hot water but continue to stir for a couple of minutes,
finally adding the lemon juice a teaspoonful each time. Season
with organic sea salt and pepper.**

To assemble
Lightly spread toast with butter or ghee (optional) or mashed avocado
and place on serving platters. Top each slice with a slice of smoked

salmon, then poached egg. Decoratively drizzle hollandaise sauce over and garnish with parsley and/or lemon wedges.

- An alternative to hollandaise sauce is to use mayonnaise to which has been added a little more lemon juice or lime juice to taste. Gently warm the mayonnaise before serving.
- In place of toasted rice bread or damper, have ready some plain fritters. Use recipe in Breads and Damper section.

Scrambled Eggs with Smoked Salmon

4 organic free range eggs
1/3 cup water
2 tablespoons chopped parsley
2 tablespoons chopped chives
Dash Herbamare herbal salt or organic sea salt
Grind fresh pepper (optional)
Butter, ghee or cold pressed oil
Slices of toasted damper, rice bread or plain fritters
2 - 4 slices smoked salmon cut into strips

Melt butter/ghee or oil in pan over medium heat to grease the pan. In a bowl, whisk together eggs, water, parsley, chives, salt and pepper and pour into the pan. Gently stir till almost set then remove and sit aside for a couple of minutes to allow it to finish cooking. Meanwhile, place hot damper, rice cake or corn cake on serving plates, spoon on scrambled egg and decorate with curls of smoked salmon. Serves 2.

- For more servings allow 2 eggs per person and a little extra water
- For an exotic taste to impress, in place of water use coconut cream or milk, and chopped coriander to replace parsley.

LUNCH

Open Sandwich - Grain-free

Sandwich base
1 medium eggplant sliced approx.2 cm/ ¾ in thick
Brown rice flour or cornmeal
Cold pressed olive oil
Organic sea salt

Topping suggestions
- Salsas on lettuce (see Salsa recipes)
- Lettuce, tomato slices, onion slices, grind of pepper, sprinkle of fresh herbs eg chopped basil, parsley or thyme
- Lettuce, sprouts, mango slices, avocado slices and slice of smoked salmon, add a dollop of homemade mayonnaise with capers, garnish with sprigs of mint

Sprinkle eggplant slices with salt and set aside for about half an hour. Rinse the slices and pat dry. Heat olive oil in fry pan, dip eggplant in brown rice flour or cornmeal and fry in the oil till golden. Drain, place on individual serving plates, 2 slices per person as for an open bread sandwich then top with any of the suggestions above.

*This open sandwich without slices of bread can be served with any gourmet sandwich topping.

Spaghetti Salad

375gms / 12oz rice spaghetti or rice/corn spaghetti cooked according to directions
12 plum tomatoes cut into chunks
1 bunch basil leaves torn into pieces
2 shallots finely chopped
¼ cup cold pressed olive oil
2 tablespoons fresh lime or lemon juice
Dash Herbamare herbal salt or sea salt (optional)
Grind of pepper (optional)

Place cooked spaghetti in a serving bowl. Toss through the tomato, basil and shallots. Combine oil, juice, salt and pepper in a jar and shake well. Add this to the salad and lightly toss. Serves 4.

- Excellent for lunch boxes
- Sprinkle with pine nuts or other chopped nuts.

Smoked Salmon Salad Stack
With Zucchini Fritters

Zucchini Fritters
2 zucchini grated
1 small onion finely chopped
2 eggs lightly beaten
¼ cup water
2-3 tablespoons brown rice flour
1 tablespoon cornflour, potato flour or arrowroot
¼ teaspoon herbal salt or sea salt
1 tablespoon chopped coriander (optional)
Grind fresh pepper
Cold pressed olive oil

Add water to egg, stir in salt, pepper and both flours to make a medium batter. To this batter add the zucchini and onion. Have ready a pan over medium heat to which has been added the olive oil and spoon in good tablespoons of mixture. When fritters appear nearly cooked (bubbles appear) turn with spatula to lightly brown the other side. Remove and drain on crumpled kitchen paper. Keep warm.

Salad Stack
4 slices of smoked salmon
Mixture of salad greens eg rocket/arugula, mizuna, beetroot greens, spinach shredded
Slices of fruit eg mango, kiwi fruit, pineapple thinly sliced
Grated carrot with a squeeze of lime
Salad onion sliced into rings
Home made mayonnaise or Lime and Coconut Dressing (see Dressings and Mayonnaise)
Sprigs of coriander or parsley

To Assemble
Place zucchini fritter on an individual serving platter. Top with the shredded salad greens, a slice of smoked salmon, grated carrot, onion

rings and sliced fruit. Drizzle with mayonnaise or Lime and Coconut Dressing, and garnish with coriander or parsley.

- The zucchini cakes can be made and placed in lunch boxes for children or adults.
- They're also delicious flavoured with homemade curry powder or a combination of ½ teaspoon each of ground coriander and cumin. Gently heat the spices or curry powder in a pan for a minute or so to release their fragrance before adding to zucchini mixture
- Alternatively, stack can be served on corn fritters. Recipe follows.
- Delicious for dinner at night

Corn Fritters

½ cup brown rice flour
1 tablespoon potato flour
1 tablespoon arrowroot or cornflour
½ teaspoon baking powder
1 large egg
1/3 cup filtered water
2 cobs of fresh sweet corn
2 shallots and green tops sliced
2 tablespoons fresh coriander or parsley chopped
¼ teaspoon Herbamare herbal salt or organic sea salt
Grind of fresh pepper (optional)
2 tablespoons cold pressed olive, sunflower, safflower or macadamia
oil

**First take a sharp knife and trim the corn from the cob and put
aside. Sift together the flours and baking powder three times to
distribute baking powder evenly. Place egg, water, salt and pepper
into a bowl and whisk lightly. Sift in dry ingredients and stir to
form a thick batter. Add corn, shallots and coriander and gently
combine. Heat pan on medium heat with the oil and place in
generous tablespoons of mixture. Cook on one side till lightly
brown then with a spatula turn to cook the other side. Serve
hot with a sauce eg a tomato sauce on a bed of rocket/arugula
surrounded by tomato wedges or alternatively serve with salsa.
(See Salsas)**

- Can be served as a stack as with Zucchini Fritters
- Excellent served cold in children's or adult's lunch box
- Serve for breakfast, perhaps with a poached egg or two on top.
- Substitute coriander with basil or herbs of your choice
- For a different flavour add fresh or dried tarragon

Mini or Large Pizzas

Small pizza bases (see recipe in Miscellaneous) or slices of gluten free bread eg rice
    bread or damper
Tomato Herb Sauce (see recipe Dressings, Mayonnaise and Sauces section)
Zucchini thinly sliced
Tomato sliced
Onion thinly sliced
Capsicum/pepper finely chopped
Olives, capers (rinsed in filtered water) or anchovies to garnish

Place bases or bread slices on baking tray, (for bread drizzle over a little cold pressed olive oil) then spread over the tomato sauce and arrange sliced and chopped vegetables on top. Garnish as desired. Bake in moderate oven 15 - 20 minutes.

Parsnip Fritters

2 medium parsnips peeled and grated
1 small onion finely chopped
1 tablespoon parsley finely chopped
¼ - ½ teaspoon Herbamare herbal salt
Dash of fresh ground pepper
1 egg
1-2 tablespoons of vegetable stock or water
1 tablespoons of potato flour
1 tablespoon of either arrowroot, cornflour or rice flour
Cold pressed olive oil

**Beat together the egg and water and blend in flours, salt
and pepper. Mix in the parsnip, onion and parsley and stir
thoroughly. Heat oil in a fry pan on medium heat and place in
tablespoons of the parsnip mixture. Gently cook for about 5
minutes on each side. These can be served hot or cold. Great to
put in a lunch box.**

- For a different flavour try 2 teaspoons home made curry powder
  in mixture.

Egg Rolls

Rolls (allow 2 eggs per person)
4 eggs
¼ cup water
Dash Herbamare herbal salt

**Whisk together eggs, water and herbal salt until just beaten.
Over beating causes egg to be tough. Pour half the mixture into
a moderately hot, greased fry pan and allow to gently set. Top
with filling of your choice, roll up and carefully lift from the pan.
Repeat with the remaining egg mixture and filling.**

Filling
1 avocado cubed
1 shallot and green top finely sliced
1 cup shredded lettuce leaves
1 medium carrot grated
½ cup bean sprouts or other sprouts
2 sprigs fresh dill chopped - extra for garnish

**Toss lightly altogether in a bowl and roll up in egg roll. Place on a
platter and garnish with extra dill. Serves 2.**

- Drizzle with some Tomato Herb Sauce either inside or over the
  roll on the platter
- Great served cold on picnics or in lunch boxes

Prawn and Avocado Roll

Egg rolls (allow 2 eggs per person)
8 eggs
½ cup water
¼ teaspoon Herbamare herbal salt

Make as for Egg Rolls above.

Filling
500gms / 1lb fresh cooked and peeled prawns
2 avocados cubed
½ red capsicum/pepper sliced
½ green capsicum/pepper sliced
3 shallots and green tops shredded
1 cup Tomato Herb Sauce or home made mayonnaise
Dash Tabasco sauce (optional)
Tomato wedges
Lettuce leaves shredded

**In a bowl gently combine prawns, avocado, capsicum and shallots.
Add the dash of Tabasco sauce to the Tomato Herb Sauce or
mayonnaise and lightly toss it through prawn and avocado filling.
Spread onto egg roll and carefully roll up. Serve on a bed of
lettuce with tomato wedges. Should make 4 rolls.**

* These rolls are also excellent as a main meal with a suitable tomato
  / lettuce salad to accompany it.

Oriental Rolls

1 cup of small broccoli florets
½ cup shallots shredded save the green tops for garnish
2 avocados cubed
2/3cup cashew nuts chopped
½ red capsicum/pepper sliced into strips
1 cup home made mayonnaise
1 small piece fresh ginger squeezed through garlic press
1 tablespoon fresh coriander or parsley finely chopped
1 teaspoon honey (optional, or date mixture see Miscellaneous)
Fresh alfalfa or snow pea sprouts/mange tout

To the mayonnaise add crushed ginger, coriander and honey and set aside for flavour to develop. In a bowl combine broccoli, shallots, cashew pieces, avocado and capsicum/pepper. Lightly toss through the mayonnaise and place filling on the cooked egg mixture and roll up. Serve on platters decorated with sprouts and green shallot tops cut into strips to form curls. Will make 4 – 6.

Avocado Omelette

4 large organic eggs
1 large avocado sliced
1 tablespoon lemon, lime or orange juice
2 tablespoons filtered water
Olive pieces or anchovies to taste (optional)
1 tablespoon fresh coriander chopped
Dash Herbamare herbal salt
Grind of pepper (optional)
Cold pressed oil for pan

**Gently toss the avocado with the juice and set aside. Lightly beat
the eggs, water, salt and pepper then add coriander. Heat and
coat a medium sized pan with the oil then pour in egg mixture
to cover the bottom of the pan. Top the omelette mixture with
sliced avocado, olives or anchovies if desired and cook over cool
to medium heat till nearly set. Place under grill to just brown the
top. Serve in wedges with an appropriate salad. Serves 2.**

- Excellent served on platters drizzled with Tomato Herb Sauce (see
  Sauce section)
- In place of olives or anchovies use capers that have been rinsed in
  filtered water.

Eggplant Rolls

1 large eggplant 1cm / ½in thick slices
Fine organic sea salt
Brown rice flour or cornmeal
Cold pressed olive oil
Fresh topping or filling of choice

Sprinkle eggplant slices with salt and set aside. After 30 minutes rinse the salt off and pat the slices dry. Coat the slices with brown rice flour/cornmeal and quickly brown both sides in a little olive oil in a fry pan. Remove and drain on kitchen paper. Spread the eggplant slices with sauces and toppings or filling of choice, roll up and secure with cocktail sticks. Place in an ovenproof dish and cook in the oven for about 15 minutes. Serve for lunch with a complementary salad.

- Can be served as finger food or entrée for dinner. Serve drizzled with a Tomato and Basil Sauce or Tomato Herb Sauce (see Sauces).
- Can be served in lunch boxes.

Homemade Bestmade Hot Potatoes

4 medium to large organic, non-GM potatoes scrubbed (but always in their jacket) and
  pricked with a fork

Fillings
- Smoked salmon cut into strips, diced avocado, diced mango and homemade mayonnaise with added lime juice and grated lime rind. Garnish with chopped fresh coriander on top. Mango can be replaced by diced fresh peaches or nectarines.
- Shredded lettuce, chopped tomato, diced cucumber, finely diced onion or shallot, finely chopped parsley, grated beetroot and a dollop of homemade mayonnaise.
- Shredded lettuce topped with any of the salsas, especially Salsa Mexicana or Spicy Pineapple Salsa all topped with a good dollop of homemade mayonnaise.

Roast potatoes on the rung of a moderate oven for about 45 minutes, or until cooked through when tested with a skewer. Remove potatoes from the oven, cut a cross on top and open out like petals to take the filling. Serve on plates with a complementary salad. Rather than roast the potatoes they can be cooked in a minimum amount of water in a saucepan (but to me they're not as nice). Serves 4.

Tacos

8 taco shells
4 cups shredded lettuce
8 hard boiled eggs chopped
Salsa of your choice
Homemade mayonnaise

Heat taco shells in oven. Fill with lettuce, eggs, salsa and top with homemade mayonnaise. A spicy salsa and/or smoked salmon or anchovies add zest to this meal. Serves 4.

• For extra special treat, omit eggs and replace with chopped, cooked, organic chicken.

Corn and Avocado Tacos

Taco shells warmed in the oven
3 fresh young cobs corn
2 avocados cubed
4 lettuce leaves shredded
1 cup grated carrot
3 shallots chopped
1 cup alfalfa sprouts, snow pea/mange tout or other sprouts
1 tablespoon parsley chopped
1 cup home made mayonnaise
1 clove garlic crushed
Dash Tabasco sauce
Tomato wedges
Dash paprika

**Combine mayonnaise, garlic and Tabasco sauce and set aside for
flavour to develop.
With a sharp knife cut corn kernels from the cob then in a large
bowl toss lightly together the corn kernels, avocado, grated carrot,
shallots and parsley. Take taco shells and place shredded lettuce
in each one. Spoon in avocado and corn mixture, then sprouts on
top. Pour on mayonnaise and sprinkle with a touch of paprika.
Serve decoratively on plates with tomato wedges. Serves about 4.**

- In place of mayonnaise, garlic and Tabasco sauce top with Tomato
  Herb Sauce (see recipe Mayonnaises, Dressings and Sauces)
- This filling is excellent in egg rolls or served as a salad.

Tortillas Mexicana (Lunch or Dinner)

¾ cup cornmeal (brown rice flour for those unable to tolerate corn)
¼ cup almond meal or macadamia nuts finely crushed
1 teaspoon fresh ground cumin heated in a pan for minute or so to
release fragrances
¼ cup vegetable stock

**In a bowl, mix together all the above ingredients then knead
until well combined. Make into about 6 even patties and roll out
between waxed lunch wrap. You should be able to get them rolled
out into thin circles. Peel off the top layer of lunch wrap and set
aside in a warm dry spot to dry out. Best done the day before or
atleast 8 hours previous. Remove and place on serving platters.**

Topping
Top with shredded lettuce greens, fresh grated carrot, sliced tomatoes,
fresh onion rings and thin rounds of fresh pineapple then a large
dollop of Chunky Guacamole (see Soups and Starters) and a side
serve of Salsa Mexicana (see Salsas)

DINNER

Soups and Starters

Pumpkin Soup with a Twist

750gms / 1½lb pumpkin peeled and chopped into chunks
1 small onion chopped
1 cup water
1 cup fresh orange juice
2-3 teaspoons grated orange rind
1 cup coconut milk
¼ teaspoon Herbamare herbal salt or sea salt
1 teaspoon ground coriander
1 teaspoon ground cumin
½ teaspoon ground cardamom
3 tablespoons cold pressed olive oil or macadamia oil
Chopped coriander or mint for garnish

Heat oil in a heavy pan and add pumpkin. Brown in the oil for about 10 minutes stirring often then add onion and gently cook till soft. Add spices and allow to heat for about a minute or so longer to allow the release of their fragrances. Pour on water, add salt and orange rind, cover and simmer until the pumpkin is tender. Allow to cool a little. Puree or whip in a blender with the orange juice. Just before serving add coconut cream and heat through. Don't boil. Serve in a soup tureen or individual serving bowls. Decorate with chopped coriander or mint. Serves 4.

- In place of ground coriander, cumin and cardamom replace with a level teaspoon of allspice and stir in chopped mint with coconut milk before serving.

Avocado Soup

2 avocadoes peeled
2 cups strong vegetable stock or fresh vegetable juice
Juice ½ lemon
Herbamare herbal salt to taste
Grind of fresh pepper (optional)
Dash Tabasco sauce (optional)
Sprigs of parsley finely chopped

Mash the avocadoes and slowly stir in the vegetable stock. Add the lemon juice and seasonings to taste. Ladle into serving bowls and garnish with chopped parsley. Serves 4.

Parsnip Soup

2 large parsnips peeled and diced
4 cups strong vegetable stock
1 tablespoon home made curry powder
3 tablespoons cold pressed macadamia, sunflower, safflower or olive oil
1 clove garlic crushed
Sprigs of Italian (flat-leafed) parsley or coriander chopped

Heat the oil in a pan over medium heat and cook the parsnip for about 5 to 10 minutes. Add the garlic and allow to gently cook for a couple of extra minutes. If cooked to long it will be bitter. Sprinkle in the curry powder and stir around for another minute to allow the release of the fragrances of the spices. Blend in the vegetable stock, cover and simmer for 30 to 45 minutes. Ladle into individual bowls or a soup tureen and sprinkle with chopped parsley or coriander. Serves 4.

Tomato and Capsicum/Pepper Soup

500gms / ½lb tomatoes peeled and chopped
2 onions sliced
2 red capsicums/pepper sliced into strips
1 cup celery diced
8 cups strong vegetable stock (see Miscellaneous)
1/3 cup cold pressed olive oil
3 eggs beaten well
Dash of Herbamare herbal salt
Fresh ground pepper (optional)
Slices of damper (see Bread section) or gluten-free bread eg rice bread
Cold pressed olive oil
Roasted knobs of garlic*

Heat the oil in a large pan and gently fry the onions till soft. Add capsicum/pepper, celery and tomatoes. Stir over medium heat for about 5 minutes then add the vegetable stock. Season to taste with salt and pepper. Cook for another 20 - 30 minutes. Remove the soup from the stove, take a couple of tablespoonsful of soup and add to beaten egg mixture, stirring it quickly. Pour back into soup, again stirring quickly so egg does not curdle. Ladle into soup bowls or tureen. Serve with slices of warm damper over which each individual can pour a little cold pressed olive oil and spread with roasted cloves of garlic. Serves 6.

* To roast the garlic, place whole knobs of garlic on shelf in a moderate oven for about 15 - 20 minutes. Cloves will cook and be spreadable.

Super Borsch

5 cups of vegetable stock (see Miscellaneous)
2 beetroot - 1 grated or julienned, 1 juiced in a juicer just before serving
1 carrot grated or julienned
1 turnip or swede/rutabaga grated or julienned
Juice of ½ lemon
Grind of fresh pepper (optional)
Chives chopped for garnish

To the vegetable stock add grated / *julienned beetroot, carrot, turnip, lemon juice and pepper. Just before serving, add beetroot juice then ladle into bowls or a soup tureen. Garnish with chives. Serves 6.
*To julienne vegetables is to cut into matchstick like sticks

- In place of lemon juice add 1½ cups of fresh orange juice before serving
- Not only is beetroot a wonderful liver tonic it is also very sweet.
- For more nutrition replace cooked stock with fresh vegetable juice.

Cucumber Soup

1 cucumber finely diced
1 cup fresh tomato juice or puree
4 cups vegetable stock
1 tablespoon chopped mint and extra sprig or sprigs for garnish
Dash Herbamare herbal salt
Grind of fresh pepper (optional)
3 eggs hardboiled and chopped
1 clove garlic
Dash Tabasco sauce (optional)
Sprig of mint

Rub the inside of a large bowl with cut clove of garlic. To it add the vegetable stock, tomato juice, cucumber, mint, salt and pepper and stir well. Chill for a few hours till ready to serve. To serve pour into soup tureen or individual bowls. Sprinkle around the chopped egg, and garnish with sprig of mint. Serves 4 - 6.

• For more nutrition, replace stock with fresh vegetable juice.

These cooked soups with dried beans and lentils have been included at the request of our daughter, Rebecca. We don't eat
nor agree with eating legumes but Rebecca reminded me that some people do.

Health Zinger

1 cup tomato juice
1 cup tomato puree
1 large onion sliced thinly
1 cup of soaked or cooked non-GM soybeans or other dried beans
2 tablespoons cold pressed olive oil
1 good teaspoon sweet paprika
½ teaspoon Herbamare herbal salt

Place all the ingredients into a saucepan simmer till beans are cooked. Garnish with chopped parsley or chives. Serves 4.

Vegetable and Lentil Stockpot

1½ cups of lentils, preferably red
6¼ cups vegetable stock, organic home - made chicken stock or water
3 - 4 medium potatoes diced
4 tomatoes peeled and chopped
2 medium onions
2 carrots diced
1 crushed clove of garlic
1 bay leaf
2 tablespoons of lemon juice
Herbamare herbal salt and fresh ground pepper to taste
Chopped parsley

Wash lentils and place in a pan with stock, tomatoes, potatoes, carrots, onions, garlic, and bay leaf. Bring to boil then reduce to simmer for about an hour or until lentils are soft. Skim off any scum that may be on the surface. Remove the bay leaf and add lemon juice and salt and pepper to taste. Ladle into soup bowls and sprinkle with chopped parsley. Serves 4 - 6.

Tomato Lentil Hotpot

1 cup of dried lentils, preferably green
6 tomatoes peeled and chopped
2 tablespoons cold pressed olive oil
1 finely chopped onion
1 crushed clove of garlic
1 tablespoon grated ginger
1 teaspoon turmeric
½ - 1 teaspoon chilli powder or to taste
1 teaspoon ground coriander
1 stick of cinnamon
1 ltr / 1¾ pints of vegetable or organic homemade chicken stock or water
Juice of a lemon
Herbamare herbal salt and fresh ground pepper
Chopped parsley

Boil lentils in plenty of water till tender (about 20 minutes). Drain. Heat oil in saucepan, saute` onion, garlic and ginger till soft. Add turmeric, chilli powder, coriander and cinnamon, and cook for a minute to release flavors. Add lentils, stock and tomatoes and simmer for 15 - 20 minutes. Stir in lemon juice, salt and pepper. (Remember to remove cinnamon stick). Garnish with chopped parsley. Serves 4.

Vegetable Stockpot

2 cups cooked organic non-GM soybeans*
2 cups tomatoes peeled and roughly chopped
½ cup chopped celery
4 tablespoons finely chopped onion
½ teaspoon Herbamare herbal salt or organic salt
1 cup water
Chopped parsley

Combine all but the parsley in a saucepan and simmer for 20 minutes. Serve garnished with chopped parsley. Serves 4.

*Soybeans should be soaked for 6 hours, rinsed in a sieve and have fresh water put on them once again and soaked for another 6 hours. This will improve the digestion of the soybeans.

Fresh Tomato Soup

5 cups fresh tomato juice or tomatoes peeled and pureed
½ salad onion finely chopped
2 cloves garlic crushed
1 tablespoon chili minced or to taste
Juice of ½ lemon
1/3 cup fresh coriander, chopped

Mix all ingredients together and refrigerate till required. Serves 4.

Carrot Soup

3 cups fresh carrot juice
1 cup of nuts, almonds or pecans, finely ground
1 cup coconut cream or thick nut milk (see Miscellaneous)
2 egg yolks
1 tablespoon cold pressed olive oil
Juice of ½ lemon or a lime
1 clove garlic crushed
2 shallots or spring onions chopped
½ red capsicum/pepper
Chopped parsley
2 teaspoons of vegetable bouillon powder

Combine nuts, coconut cream or nut milk, egg yolks, garlic lemon or lime juice, olive oil and seasoning in a blender or food processor. While still blending, slowly add the juice till all well mixed. Serve in bowls and sprinkle with chopped shallot, parsley and red capsicum/ pepper. Serves 4.

Red Soup

10 carrots
2 beetroots
4 medium tomatoes, peeled
1 small bunch of celery
½ cup raw almonds
1 tablespoon fresh thyme
1 tablespoon fresh basil
Juice of 1 lemon
Chives chopped

Juice the carrots, beetroot and celery and add lemon juice. Blend tomatoes, almonds, thyme and basil. Stir into juice and serve in bowls sprinkled generously with chopped chives.

Gazpacho

3 tomatoes, peeled
2 small cucumbers
1 tablespoon finely chopped onion
1 red capsicum/pepper chopped
3 egg yolks
3 tablespoons lemon juice
3 tablespoons cold pressed olive oil
1 clove of garlic crushed
½ cup tomato juice
2 shallots or spring onions
Dash of Herbamare herbal salt
Fresh parsley and basil chopped
1 teaspoon honey (optional)

Puree tomatoes, 1 cucumber, onion and capsicum/pepper in blender or food processor. Add the egg yolks, lemon juice, olive oil, garlic, tomato juice and honey. Finely chop the second cucumber, shallots and herbs and add just before serving. Pour into bowls and sprinkle with chopped tops of shallots or spring onions.

Rockmelon/Cantaloupe Soup

3 cups fresh pineapple or apple juice
1 cup fresh coconut milk or tinned/canned coconut cream, or organic rice milk
2 cups rockmelon/cantaloupe balls
Chopped mint
Crushed almonds, pecans or both

Blend together the juice and coconut or rice milk. Add the rockmelon/cantaloupe balls and serve in a tureen or bowls garnished with mint and nuts. Serves 2.

Watermelon and Pineapple Soup

1 cup fresh pineapple juice
2 cups pineapple finely chopped
1 cup watermelon juice
2 cups watermelon balls
Lemon or lime juice to taste
Chopped mint leaves

In a tureen or jug, gently mix together all ingredients but the chopped mint. Pour into bowls and sprinkle chopped mint on top.

Strawberry Soup

2 punnets / 8oz of strawberries
½ cup raw cashew pieces
2½ cups organic rice milk or coconut milk or nut milk (see Miscellaneous)
½ teaspoon ginger
½ teaspoon nutmeg
Sprigs of fresh mint

Blend all the ingredients but the strawberries and mint, in a blender or food processor and beat till smooth. Add strawberries and process a little longer. Serve in bowls and garnish with sprigs of mint.

Peach Soup

4 ripe peaches skin and seed removed
1 cup purified water
2 tablespoons lemon or lime juice
Grated rind of lemon or lime and half orange
Sprigs of mint
Sprinkle of nutmeg

Blend together all the ingredients but mint and nutmeg. Serve chilled in soup bowls and garnish with a sprinkle of nutmeg and sprig of mint.

- For a variation, add finely chopped chilli, finely chopped red capsicum/pepper, and sprinkle with chopped green shallot tops or chives.

Tomato Citrus Soup

2½ cups fresh tomato juice
¾ cup fresh orange juice
1 tablespoon fresh chives chopped
1 heaped tablespoon fresh dill chopped
Sprinkle of Herbamare herbal salt
Sprinkle of fresh ground pepper

Combine tomato juice, orange juice, chives, dill and seasonings. Chill till ready to serve. It should serve 4 - 6 people.

Tomato Asparagus Soup

2 cups of fresh tomato puree
1 bunch fresh crisp asparagus, tips removed and set aside, remainder
roughly chopped
2 stalks of celery
½ cup almonds ground
Small sprig oregano, leaves chopped
Small sprig basil leaves chopped
Small sprig thyme leaves stripped from stem
Dash Herbamare herbal salt (optional)

Blend together the tomato puree, chopped pieces of asparagus, celery, ground almonds, herbs and salt. Pour into a soup tureen or individual bowls and garnish with reserved asparagus tips.

Tomato and Avocado Soup

4 tomatoes peeled and roughly chopped
1 large or 2 small ripe avocadoes roughly chopped
1 stalk of celery finely chopped
1 large carrot grated
2 cups vegetable stock (see Miscellaneous) or fresh vegetable juice
2 large cloves garlic crushed
Dash Herbamare herbal salt
2 tablespoons chopped chives
Sprigs of parsley

Blend together the tomatoes, avocado, vegetable stock/juice, garlic and herbal salt. Stir in celery, carrot and chives. Serve in bowls garnished with small parsley sprigs.

Raw Carrot Soup

1 cup grated carrot
3 cups vegetable stock (see Miscellaneous) or fresh vegetable juice
½ cup almonds ground
3 shallots finely chopped
½ cup fresh chopped Italian parsley or coriander
½ teaspoon Herbamare herbal salt or organic sea salt
Chives chopped to garnish

Blend together the carrot, vegetable stock/juice, almonds and salt and pour into a bowl. Stir in shallots and parsley. Serve in individual bowls or soup tureen garnished with chopped chives.

Fresh Carrot Soup

2 cups fresh grated carrot
½ capsicum/pepper finely chopped
½ cup small broccoli florets
½ cup finely chopped celery
1 small Spanish onion finely chopped
1 cup fresh carrot juice
1 cup fresh apple juice
1 clove garlic crushed
Dash paprika to taste
1 tablespoon chopped Italian parsley or coriander

Combine all the ingredients except parsley, in a bowl. Stir well, then pour into soup tureen or individual bowls. Garnish with chopped parsley or coriander.

Vegetable Soup

1 cup finely shredded cabbage
1 small Lebanese cucumber finely diced
1 stick celery finely diced
2 shallots finely chopped, reserve green tops and shred them
½ cup sliced snow peas/mange tout
2 tomatoes peeled
1 clove garlic crushed
2 cup vegetable stock (see Miscellaneous) or fresh vegetable juice
1 teaspoon mix of herbs eg thyme, oregano and rosemary finely chopped
Dash Herbamare herbal salt

Place cabbage, cucumber, celery, shallots and snow peas in a bowl. Blend together tomatoes, garlic, vegetable stock/juice, herbs and herbal salt. Pour liquid over chopped vegetables in the bowl. Garnish with shredded green shallot tops.

Vegetable Chowder

2 cups zucchini grated
1 carrot grated
1 small Spanish onion finely diced
½ red capsicum/pepper finely diced
1 large tomato peeled and pureed
1 cup vegetable stock (see Miscellaneous) or fresh vegetable juice
1 cup fresh carrot juice
1 cup fresh orange juice
1 clove garlic crushed
1 tablespoon fresh chopped mint
Dash Herbamare herbal salt

In a large bowl or soup tureen place the chopped zucchini, carrot, onion and capsicum/pepper. Blend the tomato puree, vegetable stock/juice and garlic. Add carrot juice, orange juice and salt, just mixing to combine. Pour liquid over the chopped vegetables in the bowl and stir. Sprinkle with the chopped mint and allow to sit awhile before serving so that the flavours can mingle.

Green Pea Soup

2 cups fresh young peas
1 cup grated fresh carrot
1 medium zucchini grated
1 ripe avocado roughly chopped
2 cups vegetable stock (see Miscellaneous) or fresh vegetable juice
½ cup fresh carrot juice
Juice and rind of ½ lime
Dash Herbamare herbal salt or organic sea salt
1 tablespoon fresh dill chopped

In a bowl, combine the peas, grated zucchini and carrot. Blend together avocado, vegetable stock/juice, carrot juice, lime juice and rind and salt. Pour over other vegetables and stir. Serve in a soup tureen or individual bowls garnished with chopped dill.

Pumpkin and Pine Nut Soup

1 kg / 2lb butternut pumpkin peeled and chopped, seeds removed
2 large potatoes peeled or scraped and chopped
1 onion chopped
2 cloves garlic crushed
1 stick celery sliced
¼ cup fresh sage leaves chopped
1 tablespoon cold pressed olive oil
2 ltrs/1¾ pints vegetable stock (see Miscellaneous) or fresh vegetable juice
Fresh ground pepper (optional)
½ cup pine nuts

Heat the oil in a large saucepan and gently cook the onion, then the garlic briefly. Remember that garlic if cooked too long will taste bitter. Pour in the vegetable stock/juice, pumpkin, potatoes and celery and bring to the boil. Simmer till the vegetables are soft. Remove from heat and mash or puree the pumpkin and potato then return to the pan. Add the chopped sage, the pine nuts and if desired the pepper, and gently heat through. Serve with a damper. Serves 4 - 6.

Parsnip and Carrot Soup Morocco

2 medium-large parsnips peeled and chopped
5 carrots chopped
1 large onion chopped
2 cloves garlic crushed
2 tablespoons cold pressed olive oil or macadamia nut oil
2 teaspoons fresh ground coriander
5 cups vegetable stock (see Miscellaneous) or fresh vegetable juice
½ cup almond meal or finely crushed macadamia nuts
½ cup Italian parsley chopped
¼ teaspoon Herbamare herbal salt or organic sea salt
Grind of pepper (optional)
Curls of fresh coconut or coconut cream to serve

Heat the oil in a large saucepan and gently cook the onion until soft. Add the garlic and coriander and cook for about a further minute to release the fragrances. Next put in the chopped parsnip and carrot for another 5 minutes, frequently stirring round to slightly brown. Pour in vegetable stock, add salt and pepper and bring to the boil. Cover pan and simmer till parsnip and carrot is tender. Stir in crushed nuts and Italian parsley then blend or puree until soup is smooth. Gently reheat, then ladle soup into a pottery soup tureen or individual bowls and garnish with curls of fresh coconut, or dollop with a small spoonful of coconut cream. Serves about 4.

Hunza Soup

3 cobs fresh corn kernels cut from the cob
1 cup cucumber finely diced
1 cup fresh peas
1 large tomato finely chopped
½ cup chopped shallots including green tops
½ cup fresh asparagus tips
½ cup red capsicum/pepper finely diced
½ cup silverbeet/spinach finely shredded
1 tablespoon parsley finely chopped
1 tablespoon mint finely chopped
4 cups vegetable stock (see Miscellaneous) or fresh vegetable juice
Clove garlic crushed
¼ cup chopped almonds

**In a large bowl or soup tureen, combine all the vegetables, cover
and refrigerate till ready to serve. Add crushed clove of garlic
to the vegetable stock/juice then pour over the vegetables in the
soup tureen. Sprinkle on the finely chopped nuts and serve.
Alternatively, spoon the vegetables into individual serving bowls
then ladle over vegetable stock/juice. Garnish with nuts. This
can be served with Chapattis (see Breads, Damper, Scones and
Fritters).**

- Other vegetables of your choice can go into this soup or add more
  tomatoes.
- Add home made curry powder for a different flavour.

Simple Sushi

Cashew Sauce
2 tablespoons cashew nut butter
½ onion finely chopped
1 tablespoon cold pressed sesame, safflower, sunflower or macadamia oil
½ cup coconut milk
Pinch of chilli powder

Heat the oil in a saucepan and gently fry onion till soft. Stir in the nut butter and chilli powder, then gradually coconut milk to form a thick sauce. This needs to be thick so it doesn't run off the nori sheet. Set aside till needed.

Sushi Rolls
6 nori sheets (dried seaweed sheets)
2 cups cooked brown rice
½ teaspoon tamari (be sure it's yeast-free, gluten-free)
Juice of a lemon
1 large avocado sliced, mango sliced, prawn or strips of smoked salmon

Combine rice, tamari and lemon juice. Lay the nori (seaweed sheets) on a chopping board and using a pastry brush lightly brush over with lemon juice then spread a thin layer of the sauce to ¾ of the sheet. Next evenly spread on a layer of rice, and down the middle place a line of avocado or mango slices, prawns or smoked salmon. Roll nori sheet into a roll and leave to sit for 15 - 30 minutes. With a very sharp knife cut each roll into 3 small rolls. Serve on a platter decorated delicately with fresh nasturtium flowers or similar blossoms.

- Great in lunch boxes.

Avocado Pate

2 avocadoes flesh scooped out
4 hard boiled eggs chopped
¼ cup home made mayonnaise
2 cloves garlic
Juice of half lemon
2 sprigs mint chopped, extra sprigs reserve for garnish
Dash Herbamare herbal salt
Grind of fresh pepper (optional)
Dash paprika

**Blend or mash all the ingredients, except mint for the garnish.
Heap pate into 4 individual serving bowls, garnish with mint and
serve with corn chips or rice crackers.**

Avocado and Prawn Pate

2 avocadoes mashed with lemon juice
Juice of half lemon
300gms / ¾lb fresh prawns (reserve 8 for garnish) shelled and finely
chopped
½ cup home made mayonnaise
½ teaspoon home made mustard or Dijon mustard
Dash of paprika
Grind of fresh pepper (optional)
Sprigs of coriander or parsley and wedges of lemon to garnish

**Mash avocado, stir in lemon juice and mix together with prawns,
mayonnaise, mustard, paprika and pepper. Spoon into 4
individual pate bowls and garnish with sprigs of coriander and 2
prawns in each. Serve with lemon wedges. Serves 4.**

Chunky Guacamole

2 avocadoes
2 ripe tomatoes finely chopped
2 spring onions finely chopped
½ red capsicum/pepper finely chopped
1 red chilli finely chopped
2 cloves garlic crushed
Juice of a lime
2 teaspoons of coriander

In a glass or china bowl, mash the avocadoes, then using a wooden spoon (not metal) stir in lime juice and add remainder of ingredients. Refrigerate for an hour or so before serving. Use as a dip with fruit and vegetable sticks, corn chips, on rice crackers or toasted damper or rice bread. Serves about 4.

- Serve on plain fritters, rice or corn cakes as a topping for lunch or for the lunchbox
- Add caraway seeds to guacamole for different flavour

Avocado Asparagus Mushrooms

8 field mushrooms, stalks gently removed
4 fresh crisp asparagus spears finely chopped
1 large avocado diced
Good squeeze of lemon juice
Dash Tabasco sauce
Home made mayonnaise

Arrange mushrooms on platters. Toss asparagus with avocado, lemon juice and Tabasco. Spoon onto mushroom cups and dollop with mayonnaise. Serves 4.

A Touch of the East

2 avocadoes cubed
½ punnet / 4oz of fresh strawberries halved
2 oranges peeled, segmented and segments halved
¾ cup home made mayonnaise
1 teaspoon honey or Date Sweetener (see Miscellaneous)
½ lime juiced
1 tablespoon chopped mint leaves
Sprigs of mint for garnish

To the mayonnaise add the honey, lime juice and chopped mint leaves and set aside for the flavour to develop. In a bowl, very gently toss the avocado, strawberries and orange. Serve salad in individual bowls and just before serving dollop on the mayonnaise and decorate with mint sprigs. Serves 4.

Avocado Nests

2 avocadoes halved brushed with lemon or lime juice
2 tomatoes diced
4 shallots finely chopped
2 teaspoons basil finely chopped, reserve some basil sprigs for garnish
Macadamia nuts chopped
Cocktail Sauce (see Sauce section)

In a bowl, combine the tomatoes, shallots and basil and heap into the avocado halves. Drizzle Cocktail Sauce over and serve in avocado dishes on platters. Top with chopped macadamias and small sprigs of basil. Serves 4.

- Variations - chopped fresh mushrooms and shallots. Add some capers that have been rinsed to remove as much white vinegar as possible. Those with *Candida Albicans* beware - the mushrooms being a fungi, they may have an adverse reaction.

Fruit Cocktail
So simple, quick and refreshing

Combination of fruits cut into bite size pieces eg grapefruit, orange and mandarin segments, pineapple, peaches/nectarines, apricots, melons, cherries, quartered strawberries, peeled lychees, berries, mangoes, paw paw/papaya ... Serve in a lettuce cup or on a bed of fresh sprouts in individual bowls or glasses. Garnish with finely chopped mint or lemon balm. For an effective alternative, dip glass rims in water then into chopped mint or chives for decoration.

Asparagus and Strawberry Salad

½ bunch crisp fresh green asparagus cut diagonally into 3cm/1in pieces
½ bunch crisp fresh white asparagus cut diagonally into 3cm/ 1in pieces
1 punnet ripe strawberries quartered
3-4 cups mesclun of lettuce leaves
Mixed sprouts
Tarragon Vinaigrette Dressing (see Dressings)

Combine the asparagus and strawberries in a bowl. To serve, arrange a bed of lettuce and sprouts on individual platters or in bowls. Toss the asparagus and strawberries with the Tarragon Vinaigrette and spoon onto the bed of lettuce/sprouts on each platter. Makes an excellent first course for dinner.

Fig and Smoked Fish Platter

Fresh ripe figs quartered - allow 2 figs per person
Naturally smoked fish or eel in large bite-size pieces
Oak leaf or other lime green lettuce leaves
Alfalfa sprouts

Arrange lettuce leaves around a platter. Place fig quarters and pieces of smoked fish decoratively and alternatively in the centre. Garnish with sprouts.

- Smoked fish can be replaced with fresh cooked prawns or other seafood and served with homemade tartare sauce.

Stuffed Dried Figs

Dried figs
1 avocado mashed
1 tablespoon capers chopped, but first rinsed to remove white vinegar
Lime juice

Remove the hard stems from the figs and cut a cross on top of each one to allow it to open like the petals of a flower. Combine mashed avocado, capers and lime juice, and fill figs. Press the 'petals' back and reshape the fig. Serve as nibbles with fresh fruit cocktails.

- Try your imagination and see what delights you can make with dried figs.

Native Poi

2 cups ripe banana roughly chopped
1 tablespoon fresh lime juice
½ cup fresh coconut cream or commercial coconut cream
1 - 2 teaspoons honey (optional) or Date Sweetener (see Miscellaneous)

Puree the banana in a blender with the lime juice then slowly add the coconut cream and honey/Date Sweetener if required. Serve with pieces of fruit, coconut strips and/or pieces of vegetables.

Simple Oyster Cocktail

6 fresh oysters per person
2 tablespoons lemon or lime juice
2 tablespoons fresh tomato juice
4 tablespoons homemade mayonnaise
1 teaspoon Worcestershire Sauce
1 lettuce cup per person or torn lettuce leaves
Slices or wedges of lemon or lime

Mix together the lemon juice, tomato juice, sauce and mayonnaise. In tall cocktail glasses or small bowls place lettuce cups or torn lettuce leaves, and place fresh oysters on top. Drizzle over the cocktail sauce and serve with thin wedges of lemon/lime or with slice of lemon/lime over edge of glass.

Aioli

2 organic free range egg yolks
8 - 10 cloves garlic
1½ tablespoons fresh lemon juice
¼ teaspoon salt
1 cup approximately of good quality cold pressed olive oil

Blend together the egg yolks, garlic and salt to form a smooth paste. While blender is still running, slowly drizzle in the olive oil till only half remains, then add the lemon juice. Continue drizzling in the remaining olive oil until it is thick. Set aside till required. Serve with a platter of raw vegetable straws, florets of cauliflower and broccoli, fresh beans, sugar peas/mange tout; fruits on skewers such as avocado, grapefruit segments/other citrus.

Basil Aioli

2 organic free range egg yolks
1 cup basil leaves
4 cloves garlic crushed
1 cup cold pressed olive oil or macadamia
2 tablespoons lemon juice

Process egg yolks, garlic, basil leaves and lemon juice till smooth. While still processing, slowly add oil in a steady stream. Refrigerate aioli until required. Serve in bowl on a platter with fresh vegetable straws, broccoli and cauliflower florets, and mushrooms.

Macadamia Aioli

1 cup cold pressed olive oil
2 organic free range egg yolks
3 cloves garlic crushed
½ cup macadamia nuts finely chopped
Juice of ½ lemon or lime
2 tablespoons chives chopped
Good sprinkle Herbamare herbal salt
Fresh ground black pepper

Blend together egg yolks, garlic, lemon juice, herbal salt and pepper when well combined, while blender is still going, slowly drizzle in the oil in a steady stream until mixture thickens. Finally, by hand, fold in chopped macadamias and chives. If aioli is a little too thick add extra lemon juice. Serve in a bowl on a platter with fresh vegetable straws, broccoli and cauliflower florets, and mushrooms.

Pinzimonio

4 carrots cut into straws
1 turnip straws
1 bulb fennel straws
1 red capsicum/pepper straws/strips
1 green capsicum/pepper straws/strips
2 sticks celery straws
1 Lebanese cucumber straws
1 bunch small radishes
Anchovy Dressing (see Dressings)
Lettuce leaves

Make a bed of lettuce on a vegetable platter, leaving space in the centre for a little bowl of Anchovy Dressing. Arrange the strips of vegetables decoratively on the bed of lettuce and serve. Vegetables are dipped into dressing and eaten.

Antipasto

**Antipasto is a platter of wonderful breads and crackers,
vegetables and fruits, often pickled or marinated.
The platter is placed in the centre of the table for all to share.
Below are some suggestions for this platter.**

On a bed of lettuce serve olives, tomato wedges or cherry tomatoes, shallots with root end trimmed, but still some green top; carrot and celery straws; dried marinated tomatoes; cucumbers and chopped dill marinated in fresh lemon or lime juice; pickled cucumbers, capsicum/pepper strips, asparagus, anchovies, cold smoked fish, marinated mushrooms, slices of fresh fruit as well as fresh figs quartered. Some recipes appear below.

Bread Suggestions for Antipasto

- Take some thin slices of rice bread or damper (see Bread Section), place on an oven tray then into the oven to go crisp, dry and crunchy. Serve with your antipasto.
- To plain damper recipe, add some chopped dried tomatoes, a sprinkle of thyme, dill or chopped chives for a great savoury damper. Serve warm and sliced on the platter.
- Pop some whole knobs of garlic into a moderate oven for about 15 minutes to gently roast. Serve on the platter to spread on the slices of damper or rice bread.
- Toast some slices of rice bread to add to platter.

Pickled Cucumber

3 organic cucumbers sliced
1 small red onion thinly sliced
1 tablespoon dill finely chopped
1 lemon juiced
1 clove garlic crushed
1 teaspoon organic honey (optional)
¼ teaspoon turmeric
Good pinch cayenne
1 teaspoon Herbamare herbal salt or organic sea salt
1/3 cup filtered water

In a bowl, combine sliced cucumber, onion and dill. Mix together lemon juice, garlic, honey, turmeric and cayenne then add the salt and water. Pour this over the cucumber and onion and refrigerate for an hour or two till ready to serve on your antipasto.

- Zucchini can replace the cucumber and be served in the same way.

Marinated Vegetables

1 cup broccoli and/or cauliflower florets
1 red capsicum/pepper cut into wide strips
Fresh crisp green beans cut into halves
Crisp asparagus spears, top half only (the spear end)
½ cup good cold pressed olive oil
1/3 cup fresh lemon juice
1 teaspoon organic honey (optional)
1 clove garlic crushed
Sprig fresh oregano chopped
Sprig fresh thyme leaves stripped from stems

Place all vegetables in a large bowl. In a jar, combine the oil, honey, garlic, herbs and lemon juice and shake vigorously to combine. Pour this over the vegetables and very gently toss to coat. Cover and set aside for one to three hours atleast, gently tossing occasionally. Serve decoratively on your antipasto platter.

• You can try any vegetable that may appeal to you, strips of carrot, turnip/swede(rutabaga), use your imagination and sense of taste.

Marinated Eggplant

500gms / ½lb thin eggplants sliced diagonally, or larger eggplant
cubed
3 tablespoons good cold pressed olive oil
2 tablespoons fresh lemon juice
2 cloves garlic crushed
2 anchovy fillets finely chopped
Extra olive oil
1 tablespoon chopped parsley

**Blend together the olive oil, lemon juice, garlic and anchovies.
Set aside. Sprinkle eggplant slices with organic sea salt and leave
for about 30 minutes. Rinse the salt from the eggplant, pat slices
dry and brown both sides in extra oil in a fry pan. Place them in
a large bowl. Gently toss through the marinade, cover and allow
to sit for about 4 hours. Add parsley and serve on a platter with
other vegetables and damper or rice bread slices.**

Dried Tomatoes in Olive Oil

Dried tomatoes
Good cold pressed olive oil
Clove of garlic
1 teaspoon small capers, rinsed under water to remove white vinegar
(optional).
Fresh sprigs of thyme, rosemary, oregano and/or basil
Slightly cracked peppercorns (optional)

**Place dried tomatoes in a screw top jar alternatively with the
garlic, capers, thyme and herbs of choice and gently pour
over olive oil. Replace lid, and store in a cool dark place for a
minimum of 4 weeks when the tomatoes will be ready to serve on
an antipasto platter. The oil will have a wonderful flavour to be
used in dressings and mayonnaise.**

Bruschetta with Tomato and Basil

Slices of rice bread or damper (see Bread section) toasted
2 large cloves garlic halved or oven roasted knob of garlic
3 large ripe tomatoes finely chopped
¼ cup fresh basil leaves finely shredded
Grind of fresh pepper (optional)
Good quality cold pressed olive oil

Combine the tomato, basil and pepper in a bowl. Rub the slices of hot toasted bread/damper with cut cloves of garlic. Drizzle each slice with a little olive oil and top with the tomato and basil. Serve while hot. If using roasted cloves of garlic, drizzle first with the olive oil and spread with the garlic before adding the topping.

- Add some finely diced red capsicum/pepper to the topping.
- To garnish place 3 or 4 good black olives and small sprig of basil decoratively on each plate. Alternatively, add chopped olives or anchovies to the topping.

Dukkah and Dukkan

are coarsely ground Egyptian nut and spice blends. Serve them
in a small bowl side by side with another bowl of good quality
cold pressed olive oil. The recipes for Dukkah and Dukkan
(pronounced *dooka or dookan)* were given to me by a lovely lady
called Fay. She tells me that these mixes are used for dunking
pieces of fresh bread, first into olive oil, then dipped into the
dukkah or dukkan then eaten, and as Fay would say, "and enjoy".
This mix can also be used for sprinkling on soft-boiled eggs, for
coating salmon or other fish, or lamb (for those who eat meat),
and then char-grilled. The prepared dukkah and dukkan can be
made and stored in an airtight jar in the refrigerator ready for
use. I see its uses much more varied, we've tried them on different
foods…and believe me, it's an excellent condiment for many
simple fresh fruit and vegetable dishes.
Three recipes follow.

Dukkah 1.

8 tablespoons sesame seeds
4 tablespoons coriander seeds
3 tablespoons cumin seeds
50gms / 2oz hazelnuts
1 teaspoon organic sea salt (I make it with only ¼ teaspoon, we don't
eat lots of salt)
½ teaspoon peppercorns (can be less if wished) dry roasted - it is a
spice

In a saucepan over medium heat, briefly roast each ingredient
separately. Rub the skin from the hazelnuts before grinding. In
a spice grinder place all the roasted spices and grind. By gently
roasting them we are actually releasing their special flavours. (Fay
told me to use a coffee grinder and keep it just for grinding my
spices fresh before using them…and it works great). Grind up the
skinned hazelnuts then combine all ingredients and store in an
airtight jar in the refrigerator till needed.

Dukkah 2.

½ cup sesame seeds roasted
100gms / 4oz hazelnuts or any other nut
2 tablespoons cumin seeds
1 tablespoon ground cardamom
2 teaspoons coarse organic sea salt (optional - I use about ½ teaspoon)
2 teaspoons peppercorns

Process all ingredients in a blender until nuts are finely chopped, and mixture is well combined. Store in an airtight glass jar in the refrigerator till required.

Dukkan

½ cup sesame seeds
½ cup coriander seeds
1/3 cup cumin seeds
¼ cup almonds dry roasted and skin removed as for hazelnuts above
Organic sea salt and peppercorns as for above

As for dukkah, dry roast the sesame seeds, each of the spices (including peppercorns) and the almonds. Grind the spices and almonds then add to the sesame seeds in an airtight glass jar. Store in the refrigerator till required.

- Brush avocado halves with olive oil and lemon/lime dressing and sprinkle with any of the above. Alternatively, just use the oil and nut/spice mix, it's delicious.
- Try fruit and vegetables straws, or use your imagination and be creative.
- Coat seafood in dakkah or dakkan to char-grill.
- Dip hot pieces of damper or rice bread. Serve as an appetizer before a meal.

Curried Macadamia and Mango Dip

1 mango skin and seed removed
1 small onion chopped
1 clove garlic crushed
100gms / 2oz macadamia nuts
2 teaspoons home made curry powder
¼ cup home made mayonnaise
1 teaspoon honey or Date Sweetener (see Miscellaneous)
Dash of organic sea salt
Mint or coriander to garnish

Place all ingredients into a blender and process. Decorate with a sprig of mint or coriander. Serve with a platter of vegetable sticks and pieces of fresh fruit eg carrots, celery, cucumber, zucchini, turnip or swede/rutabaga, snow peas/mange tout or cauliflower and broccoli florets; fruits such as apple and pear slices (dipped in lemon or orange juice to prevent browning) and strawberries. Alternatively, rice crackers and/or corn chips would do nicely.

My Humus

2 cups ground nuts eg almonds, macadamias, pine nuts or mixture
¼ cup lemon or lime juice
2 cloves garlic crushed
½ teaspoon cumin seed freshly ground
Dash of Herbamare herbal salt or organic sea salt
Dash cayenne
1 tablespoon of chopped parsley or mint

Blend together all the ingredients but parsley or mint. Mix in parsley or mint last. Set aside till required and to let the flavours develop. Serve with crackers, or vegetable and fruit pieces.

*   If your taste says you need it sweetened try adding the Date Sweetener, recipe in Miscellaneous.

Quick Coconut Dip

1 cup coconut cream
Juice of lime to make thick consistency and a little grated rind
1 teaspoon fresh ground cumin seed
1 teaspoon fresh coriander seed
1 tablespoon finely chopped fresh coriander

Gently heat the coriander and cumin for a minute or two to release their fragrances. Combine all ingredients in a container and set aside for flavours to develop. Serve dip with chopped fresh pieces of fruit as an appetizer eg pineapple, orange, apple, pear, strawberries etc or alternatively, cooked prawns.

Almond Dip

½ cup almond butter
1 tablespoon fresh basil or dill finely chopped
1 clove garlic crushed
½ lime or lemon juiced and grated rind to taste
1 teaspoon organic honey, maple syrup or Date Sweetener (see Miscellaneous)
Dash Herbamare herbal salt or organic sea salt

Mix together the ingredients, adding a little filtered water if too stiff. Set aside to allow the flavours to develop. Serve with a platter of vegetables eg carrot, celery, cucumber straws, cauliflower and broccoli florets or chopped fruits.

Carrot and Ginger Dip

3 carrots roughly chopped
3 tomatoes peeled and roughly chopped
1 onion chopped
1 clove garlic crushed
2 teaspoons fresh ginger grated
1 good sprig of thyme leaves stripped from stems
1 good sprig of tarragon
¼ cup home made mayonnaise
Squeeze of lemon juice
Dash of Herbamare herbal salt or sea salt to taste
Grind of fresh pepper
Sprinkle of nutmeg

Finely mince carrots in a blender or food processor, then add onion, ginger and garlic, and process again. Blend in the tomatoes, herbs, salt and pepper and finally the mayonnaise with the squeeze of lemon. Spoon into a serving bowl and sprinkle on top with nutmeg (fresh ground would be excellent). Serve with vegetable straws and florets of cauliflower, corn chips or rice crackers.

Remoulade

½ cup homemade mayonnaise
1 tablespoon capers chopped (rinsed first in filtered water to remove
white vinegar)
2 small pickled cucumbers finely chopped
1 bunch dill chopped
1 teaspoon home made mustard or Dijon mustard
1 teaspoon apple or pear juice concentrate or Date Sweetener (see
Miscellaneous)
Dash organic sea salt
Grind fresh pepper

**Mix together all the ingredients and set aside till required. Dip in
pieces of cucumber, celery sticks, julienned (strips) turnip, carrot;
cauliflower and broccoli florets, asparagus pieces, almost any raw
vegetable. Also pieces of apple and pear will go with this dip.**

- Serve this dip as a topping over a hot potato.
- Can be used as a type of mayonnaise for salads or coleslaws.

THE MAIN EVENT

This consists of fish, raw and cooked, eggs, nuts, and sometimes for a special occasion, game or an organic chicken for the main meal. Although a number of these dishes are cooked, use these on your way to weaning yourself from lots of cooked food to raw food. You should try to eat as much raw foods as possible, as Mother Nature intended. I know we all crave cooked 'comfort foods' on occasions, but they are not meant to be eaten everyday.

Poached Trout

1 large or 2 small rainbow trout, heads and tails intact
¾ cup water
¾ cup lime or lemon juice
½ onion sliced
½ stalk celery
1 bay leaf
1 small sprig parsley
4 peppercorns
¼ teaspoon salt

Place all ingredients into pan, except trout, and bring to the boil. Gently poach trout in liquid for 5 - 6 minutes. If trout is to be eaten hot, serve on heated platter, drizzled with melted butter/ ghee or olive oil and lemon juice. To serve trout cold, allow to cool in the liquid, and when ready to be eaten carefully remove skin from tail to gills. Place on a platter and serve with Seafood Sauce (see recipe below). Serves 2

Seafood Sauce
2/3 cup home made mayonnaise
1 tablespoon tomato paste
Good squeeze of lime or lemon juice
½ teaspoon grated zest of lemon
Fresh ground black pepper

Combine all the above ingredients and when ready to serve, pour decoratively over trout. Garnish with lemon wedges.

- Alternatively, can be served with Lime and Coconut Dressing.

Oven-cooked Trout

1 - 2 trout washed, left whole
Lime slices
A little oil or butter/ghee

**Grease oven tray with oil or butter/ghee. Place trout on tray
and cover with unbleached greaseproof paper or a lid. Cook in**

**a moderate oven for about 15 minutes. On the upside of fish
gently slice skin around at the head under the gill and at tail and
peel carefully off. Place on serving platter, decorate with lime**

slices along the fish and serve with sauce of your choice.

- Serve with Lime and Coconut Dressing or Tomato Herb Sauce
- White fleshed fish tastes excellent cooked like this also.
- Spoil yourself and drizzle with Hollandaise Sauce.

Trout Almandine

1 large or 2 small trout
Brown rice flour or cornmeal
2 tablespoons butter/ghee
1 tablespoon macadamia nut oil
Chopped chives
Almond Sauce (see below)

Skin trout from tail to gills, roll in brown rice flour. Heat butter and oil in fry pan and when hot enough (it is foaming) add trout and cook for about 5 - 6 minutes, turning carefully once to allow even cooking. Check with a sharp knife at fish's thickest part to determine when cooked, then transfer to hot plates. Pour over the Almond Sauce and sprinkle with chopped chives. Serve with a light crisp salad. Serves 2.

Almond Sauce
2 tablespoons butter/ghee
¼ cup slithered almonds
1 tablespoon lemon juice
Fresh ground black pepper

Gently melt butter/ghee and add almonds, allowing them to turn just golden. Add lemon juice and pepper, pour over fish and serve.

•   Trout can be replace with Atlantic salmon fillets or cutlets.

Smoked Fish or Fish Fillets

2 - 4 fish fillets or whole fish
2 teaspoons of jasmine tea leaves

Sprinkle jasmine tea leaves into the bottom of a wok then place a round cake cooler inside. Lay fish fillets on top of cake cooler and place on the lid. Sit the wok on the hotplate, heated on low to medium heat. The tea leaves will smoke and gently cook the fish in about 8 minutes, depending on thickness of fish or fillets. Serve with a complementary salad.

Ceviche`
A Favourite

500gms / 1lb white firm-fleshed fish fillets
2 lemons or limes juiced
2 tomatoes peeled and diced small
1 small red capsicum/pepper, diced small
1 small salad onion or shallots finely chopped or sliced
4 tablespoons chopped parsley
1 avocado, cubed
1 small chilli finely chopped (optional)
Lettuce cups

Remove skin and bones from raw fish and cut into small cubes. Place in a china or glass bowl and cover with the lemon or lime juice. Leave to marinate for a minimum of 3 hours, turning the fish from time to time with a wooden or plastic spoon. Drain the juice from the fish and add the diced tomatoes, diced capsicum/ pepper, onion, parsley, oregano, chilli and avocado and spoon into serving bowls lined with the lettuce cups. Garnish with sprig of parsley. Serves 4.

Marinated Fish

2 white-fleshed fish fillets skinned
1 tablespoon cold pressed macadamia nut oil
1 tablespoon cold pressed sesame oil (use walnut, almond or olive if preferred)
Juice and grated rind of 1 orange
3 bay leaves
6 - 8 black peppercorns
Mesclun of lettuce and salsa to serve

In a screw top jar combine oils, orange juice and rind, bay leaves and peppercorns. Shake until well mixed. Place fish fillets in a shallow glass or china dish and pour over the marinade. Cover and refrigerate for minimum 12 hours up to 24 hours, turning occasionally. To serve, remove bay leaves place on platter with lettuce and salsa.

Fish in Coconut Cream

500gms / 1lb white, firm fleshed fish fillets
Juice of 3 limes, or lemons if limes are unavailable
1 red capsicum/pepper, diced small
2 shallots or spring onions, and green tops chopped
1 stalk of celery diced
½ cup coconut cream
Fresh ground black pepper
Sprinkle of Herbamare herbal salt
Lettuce cups and mixed fresh sprouts
Sprigs of parsley

Remove skin and bones from the fish and cut into cubes. Place in a china or glass bowl and pour over the lime juice. Leave to marinate for a minimum of 3 hours, turning with a wooden or plastic spoon from time to time. Drain the juice from the fish and add diced capsicum/pepper, celery and shallots. Pour on the coconut cream and toss well. Season with herbal salt and pepper. Chill. Serve in individual bowls lined with lettuce cups and sprouts. Garnish with sprigs of parsley. Serves 4.

Marinated Seafood Marquesan Style

500gms / 1lb fresh white fleshed fish cubed into 2cm/¾in pieces, or
scallops, mussels etc
1 small Spanish/red onion thinly sliced
¾ cup fresh lime juice
¼ cup fresh grated coconut

**Place fish or chosen seafood into a glass or pottery bowl and
cover with the lime juice. Marinate over night or all day, atleast
12 hours. Drain the juice and reserve for salad dressing. Add the
grated fresh coconut and serve with an appropriate salad, drizzled
with a dressing made with the reserved lime juice.**

My Sashimi

250gms / 8oz fresh tuna thinly sliced
½ cup orange oil*
2½cm/1in piece fresh ginger grated or pressed through garlic press

**Mix together the orange oil and ginger. Decoratively place tuna
slices on individual serving plates and drizzle with the oil. Serve
with a delicately flavoured salad of light green lettuce leaves, slices
of cucumber, radishes, carrot, shallot strips mandarin segments,
pear or apple slices dipped in orange juice (to prevent oxidation)
or a delicately flavoured fruit salsa .**

*To macadamia, almond, avocado or olive oil add the grated orange
rind of half an orange, and sit for 3 or 4 hours to allow the orange
flavour to develop in the oil.

Fish in Banana Leaves

6 fillets of snapper, bream or other white fleshed fish
1 large banana leaf
Juice of 2 limes

Marinade
6 shallots thinly sliced
2 cloves garlic crushed
1 red chilli finely chopped (optional)
4 stalks lemon grass
Grated rind of 2 limes
Small piece of green ginger crushed (in garlic press)
3 tablespoons cold pressed macadamia nut, sunflower, safflower or olive oil
3 tablespoons fresh pineapple juice
1 tablespoon organic honey or Date Mixture (see Miscellaneous)

Combine the ingredients of the marinade well. Place fish in a glass or china dish and marinate for 2 to 3 hours in the refrigerator. Wrap the fish up as parcels in single pieces of banana leaf, with some of the marinade added, and tie. Cook on the grill of a barbecue for about 15 minutes. Serve with a complementary salad or fresh pineapple slices and macadamia nuts on a bed of torn rocket/arugula leaves.

- Banana leaves can often be purchased in large supermarkets or whole food stores
- In place of banana leaf try using sorrel leaves, lettuce leaves, cabbage leaves etc

Spiced Fish

4 fish fillets
1 good tablespoon brown rice flour or cornmeal
2 teaspoons sweet paprika
1 teaspoon fresh ground cumin
1 teaspoon cinnamon
Cold pressed olive or macadamia oil

Mix together the dry ingredients and sprinkle over the fish fillets. Heat the oil in a frypan and gently brown fish on both sides. Continue to cook till just done. Remember, over cooked seafood is tough and dry. Serve with a salsa of your choice and an appropriate salad. Serves 4.

- Cook some banana slices with fish for a tropical touch, and squeeze lime juice or lemon over fish and banana to serve.

Baked Fish

4 fresh white fish fillets
2 cups rice breadcrumbs
3 cloves garlic crushed
3 tablespoons butter/ghee, or cold pressed olive or macadamia oil
1 tablespoon Italian parsley finely chopped
1 lemon to squeeze
Lemon wedges

Lightly oil an ovenproof dish and arrange fish across the bottom. Mix together the parsley and rice breadcrumbs, and spread over the fish fillets in the dish. If using butter/ghee, heat till just melted. Stir crushed garlic into butter/ghee or oil and drizzle over the breadcrumbs. Bake in a moderate oven for about 15 minutes until the breadcrumbs are golden brown. Remove from the oven and squeeze fresh lemon juice over the top. Serve on each plate with a lemon wedge and parsley sprig, and accompany with an appropriate salad. Serves 4.

- In place of Italian parsley try summer savoury, lemon thyme, coriander or chives.
- For added flavour, sprinkle chopped shallots over the fish and mix the finely chopped green tops in the breadcrumbs.
- To the topping add 2 tablespoons capers finely chopped (rinse first to remove the white vinegar), a grind of fresh pepper, and oil or butter/ghee replaced by a lightly beaten egg. Once again squeeze with lemon juice after cooking.

Fish Cakes with Lime and Dill

250gms / ½1lb white fish fillets cooked and flaked
1 egg
3 chopped shallots
1 tablespoon lime juice
2 teaspoons grated rind of lime
1 tablespoon fresh dill chopped
Dash Herbamare herbal seasoning salt
Fresh ground black pepper
Cold pressed olive oil or macadamia nut oil.

Process fish in food processor till smooth. In a bowl, mix fish, shallots, egg, dill, lime and seasonings. Form into 4 patties and cook in oil for 5 - 6 minutes, turning once. Drain on kitchen paper and serve with lettuce leaves, sliced tomato, sliced avocado and home made mayonnaise with capers. (See Mayonnaise recipe). Serves 2.

Grilled or Barbecued Fish with Eggplant

4 fish fillets or cutlets
Good cold pressed olive oil
1 kg / 2lb eggplant sliced and sprinkled with salt
1/3 cup cold pressed olive oil
¼ cup lemon juice
1 clove garlic crushed
Herbamare herbal salt or organic sea salt to taste
Fresh black pepper to taste (optional)
4 medium ripe tomatoes cut into wedges
Lettuce leaves
Chopped fresh parsley

Allow salt to stay on eggplant slices for about 30 minutes, then rinse in filtered water and pat dry. Brush both sides with olive oil, place on an oven tray and roast in the oven for 30 minutes. Once cooked, skin the eggplant and puree with the oil, lemon juice, garlic, salt and pepper. To cook fish fillets brush with oil and cook on grill or barbecue 3 to 4 minutes each side depending on thickness of fish. To serve, arrange lettuce leaves to the side on individual platters, top with tomato wedges and sprinkle well with parsley. Place fish in pride of place in centre of platter and spoon eggplant puree across the middle. Serves 4.

Crumbed Atlantic Salmon Cutlets

2 salmon cutlets
2 tablespoons butter/ghee
1 tablespoon cold pressed oil
2 tablespoons brown rice flour or cornmeal

In a container, place the brown rice flour or cornmeal and salmon cutlets. Make sure the lid is on firmly, then shake to coat the fish with rice flour or cornmeal. Have butter/ghee and oil heating in frypan, when frothing place in salmon cutlets and quickly cook turning once, until just cooked. As with all seafood it will become dry or tough if overcooked. Serve with a salsa, Almond Butter Sauce, Lime and Coconut Dressing or Seafood Sauce and a complementary salad. Serves 2.

Salmon and Pineapple Salad

2 medium sized salmon cutlets
1 tablespoon cold pressed good quality sesame oil or macadamia nut oil
1½ cups fresh pineapple chopped
1 Lebanese cucumber sliced diagonally
2 tablespoons fresh coriander leaves
2 tablespoons fresh mint leaves
1 red chilli seeded and finely chopped (optional)
1 stalk fresh lemon grass thinly sliced
1 kaffir lime leaf very thinly sliced
Lettuce leaves
Fresh mixed sprouts
Fresh coconut flaked or coarsely grated
Oriental Dressing (see Dressings)

Heat the oil in a pan and gently cook the salmon cutlets on both sides till just done. Don't over cook. Combine all the remaining ingredients, except dressing, in a large bowl. Flake the salmon into chunks and place in the bowl with salad. Gently toss through enough dressing to coat. Serve on lettuce leaves and sprouts in individual salad bowls and garnish with fresh coconut. Serves 4.

Scallops and Avocado

4 avocadoes halved, flesh carefully scooped out with a spoon and cubed
8 scallops halved
2 small onions finely sliced
1 apple finely diced (Granny Smith is my favourite)
1 tablespoon cold pressed macadamia, sunflower, safflower or sesame oil
½ teaspoon ground coriander
½ teaspoon ground cumin
½ teaspoon turmeric
½ cup coconut cream
¼ cup organic white wine or grape juice (check for unsweetened, preservative-free)
Fresh coriander chopped

Gently combine cubed avocado, onions and apple in a bowl. Heat the oil in a pan and sprinkle in the spices, then add the scallops. Cook for 2 minutes on medium heat. Pour on wine or grape juice and stir around. Add coconut cream and heat through, making sure mixture doesn't boil. Remove from the heat and lightly and quickly stir in avocado mixture. Spoon back into avocado halves and serve with a complementary salad eg pineapple, cucumber, mixture of lettuce, radishes etc. Can be served warm or cold. Serves 4.

Scallops or Mussels with Herbs and Garlic

20 scallops or mussels in shell (and cleaned)
2 tablespoons good cold pressed olive oil, macadamia or safflower oil
1 lime juiced
2 cloves garlic crushed
¼ cup mixed chopped herbs eg Italian parsley, oregano, basil,
coriander, lemon balm
Grind of black pepper (optional)
Lime wedges to serve

**Combine the oil, lime juice, garlic and herbs. Place the scallops
or mussels on a tray and spoon over the herb and garlic mixture.
Grind some black pepper over them and pop under the grill for 2
to 3 minutes till just opaque (cooking seafood too long will make
it tough and dry). Serve immediately with lime wedges and a
complementary salad. Serves 4.**

• This dressing of herbs and garlic will also work with fish, either
  oven baked, grilled under a grill or cooked on a barbecue. Leave
  fish to marinate for 30 to 60 minutes before cooking. In the
  oven I would check after about 10 to 12 minutes and with a
  grill or barbecue 4 to 5 minutes on both sides should see the fish
  cooked. (It will also depend on the thickness of the fish). Double
  the quantity of dressing to do 4 fish fillets or cutlets in place of
  mussels or scallops.

Marinated Scallops, Mussels or Squid (Calamari)

20 scallops, mussels or 2 squid tubes cut into rings
3-4 limes juiced
½ cup coconut cream or milk
2 avocadoes quartered and chopped
2 tomatoes chopped
1 tablespoon fresh coriander chopped
1 tablespoon chives chopped
Lettuce leaves and fresh sprouts
Lime wedges to serve

Place scallops, mussels or squid rings into a glass or ceramic bowl. Pour lime juice over the seafood and gently mix through. Allow to marinate atleast 3 hours turning frequently with a wooden spoon (no metal spoon, it will discolor seafood). Drain the seafood, add the avocado, tomato, coriander and chives then gently toss through the coconut cream or milk. Serve on individual platters, on a bed of lettuce and fresh sprouts. Serves 4.

Tropical Seafood Salad

4 cups shelled cooked prawns, crab/lobster meat, or squid tubes sliced
and poached in
  lime juice and cold pressed oil
½ pineapple peeled, cored and cut into pieces
1 mango cubed
1 cup paw paw/papaya cubes
1 avocado cubed
½ cup macadamia nuts
½ cup coconut cream or homemade mayonnaise
1 tablespoon lime juice
1 tablespoon fresh, chopped chives
Lettuce leaves
Mixed fresh sprouts

**Mix coconut cream or mayonnaise with lime juice and set aside.
In a large bowl combine seafood, pineapple, mango, paw paw/
papaya and avocado. Gently toss through the coconut cream or
mayonnaise and serve on a bed of lettuce and sprouts. Garnish
with macadamia nuts.**

• Alternative - use cold cooked fish or natural, cold smoked fish.

Pear and Salmon Cups

4 pears peeled, halved and cored, dipped in citrus to prevent browning
*Medium sized tin/can pink salmon drained
1 tablespoon homemade mayonnaise
2 shallots and green tops chopped
Teaspoon capers (rinsed under running water to remove white vinegar)
Good squeeze of lemon or lime juice
Fresh ground black pepper
1 avocado cut into fan
Alfalfa sprouts and sprigs of dill to decorate
Lettuce leaves

Combine salmon, lemon/lime juice, mayonnaise, shallots, capers and black pepper. Serve heaped on upturned pear halves, placed on a bed of lettuce. Decorate with fans of avocado, alfalfa sprouts and dill sprigs. For a variation you could serve the salmon on a bed of lettuce and sprouts, decorated with sliced pear halves and fanned avocado. Serves 2.
* In place of tinned/canned salmon, use cooked salmon cutlets or naturally smoked fish

Seafood in Fruit Cups

4 fresh pears or peaches, halved and dipped in citrus to prevent
browning
Seafood - mixture of fresh, cooked prawns, scallops, mussels, oysters
French dressing (see Dressings)
Clove of garlic crushed
Chopped sprig of parsley
Lettuce leaves

**Combine French dressing, garlic and parsley, and marinate
seafood in the dressing for about 3 hours. Place upturned pear or
peach halves on a bed of lettuce and garnish with small sprigs of
dill. Serve with a complementary salsa.**

• Can be served with Lime and Coconut Dressing.

Barbecued Fish Kebabs

500gms / 1lb fish cubed
2 red capsicums/peppers cut in large dice
1 onion cut into large dice
2 cups fresh pineapple in chunks

Marinade
½ cup cold pressed olive oil, macadamia nut oil or sesame oil
2 cloves garlic crushed
1 small onion finely chopped
1 tablespoon lemon juice
1 teaspoon honey or Date Sweetener (see Miscellaneous)
1 teaspoon home made mustard (see recipe Miscellaneous)

Combine the marinade ingredients and pour over cubed fish for minimum 1 hour. Stir around to make sure the fish is coated. Drain fish and thread alternately onto skewers with capsicum/ pepper, onion and pineapple. Have barbecue grill ready and place kebabs on. Turn frequently while basting with marinade. Should be cooked in 5 to 6 minutes. Serve with a complementary salad of your choice.

• Add fresh pieces of coconut.

Salmon and Sweet Potato Curry

500gms / 1lb sweet potato peeled and cubed
1 large tin of pink salmon
Cold pressed oil
1 large onion finely chopped
2 teaspoons fresh ginger grated / minced
1 red chilli seeded and finely chopped
1 tablespoon home made curry powder (see recipe Miscellaneous)
1 cup coconut cream
¾ cup natural organic sultanas or raisins
3 tablespoons fresh coriander chopped
Juice of a lemon or lime
Zest of lime or lemon

Heat oil in fry pan and gently fry sweet potato in oil till golden brown. Remove sweet potato to a plate then gently fry onions, ginger and chilli until onion is soft. Sprinkle in curry powder and fry for a further 1 minute to release the fragrances. Add sweet potato, sultanas/raisins, coconut cream and coriander. Place lid on the pan and simmer just long enough to cook sweet potato. Add lemon/lime juice and zest, and stir through. Serve with a complementary salad.

Quick Salmon Curry

Medium size tin of pink salmon
1 cup coconut milk
1 medium onion chopped
1 tablespoon homemade curry powder (see recipe see Miscellaneous)
1 ripe banana, apple or pear chopped
½ cup natural sultanas (optional)
Juice of lemon or lime
1 - 2 tablespoons cold pressed oil

Heat oil in a pan and gently cook onion. Add curry powder and allow to heat for about a minute to bring out flavours. Add coconut milk, salmon, banana and sultanas. Simmer gently for a further 5 minutes, add lemon juice and serve with an appropriate salad. Serves 2.

Salmon Quiche

Pie Crust
3 cups ground nuts eg almond or macadamia
1 egg yolk
2 tablespoons butter/ghee melted or cold pressed olive oil
¼ teaspoon Herbamare herbal salt or organic sea salt

Filling
1 medium can of salmon
8 anchovies in oil, drained and chopped
3 eggs
1½ cups organic rice milk or nut milk
2 tablespoons chopped parsley
½ teaspoon paprika
¼ teaspoon Herbamare herbal salt
Fresh ground black pepper

Form pie crust by combining ground nuts, egg yolk and melted butter/ghee or oil. Press into 23cm pie dish. For the filling, drain and flake the salmon, saving some liquid. Arrange salmon and anchovies evenly over the pastry base. Beat together eggs, salmon liquid, rice/nut milk, parsley, paprika, herbal salt and pepper. Pour mixture slowly over the back of a spoon onto fish so that it covers the fish without flushing it into a mound. Bake in moderate over for 40 to 45 minutes or until egg mixture is set (when a knife is inserted and comes out clean). Serves 6.

- An excellent picnic food.
- For a great taste, replace rice/nut milk with coconut milk and parsley with coriander

Hot Prawns with Cool Avocado Salsa

¾kg / 1½lb uncooked prawns shelled
2 teaspoons cold pressed olive or macadamia nut oil
2 tablespoons limes juice
2 tablespoons fresh coriander chopped
1 fresh red chilli finely chopped
2 teaspoons ground cumin
Extra cold pressed oil for frying
Lettuce leaves
Avocado Salsa (see Salsas)

Place the prawns in a glass or china bowl. Combine the oil, lime juice, coriander, chilli and cumin and pour over the prawns. Allow to marinate 10 to 15 minutes. Heat extra oil in frypan and cook for about 2 to 3 minutes, till the prawns are just red. Remember, over cooking seafood makes it tough. Serve in salad bowls lined with lettuce leaves, and complement with the Avocado Salsa. Serves 4.

Steamed Ginger Prawns with Salsa

¾kg / 1½lb green prawns shelled
5cm / 2in piece ginger thinly sliced
4 cloves garlic thinly sliced
2 tablespoons cold pressed macadamia nut oil
Lettuce leaves and fresh mixed sprouts
Salsa (see Salsas)

Heat oil in a small pan and quickly cook garlic slices till crisp and golden, (about 30 seconds) but don't burn. Set aside. Layer the base of a steamer with ginger slices, place in prawns and simmer over water for about 3 to 5 minutes, remember overcooking seafood makes it tough. Line individual salad bowls with lettuce leaves and sprouts, spoon on the prawns and add a salsa of your choice. Serves 4 to 6.

- Great served with Mango Salsa, Spiced Peach Salsa, Pineapple Salsa or Kiwi Salsa.

Prawn Salad

500gms / 1lb prawns cooked and shelled
1 cup grapes well washed
1 cup homemade mayonnaise
½ lime or lemon juiced
2 tablespoons fresh dill chopped
2 tablespoons fresh chives chopped
Fresh ground black pepper
Lettuce leaves and fresh alfalfa sprouts

Place prawns, grapes, fresh dill and chives into a bowl. Add juice and ground pepper to homemade mayonnaise then combine with other ingredients. Toss through lightly, cover and refrigerate till required. Serve in bowls lined with lettuce leaves and sprouts.

Marinated Squid

500gms / 1lb squid tubes
1/3 cup cold pressed olive oil
1/3 cup lemon or lime juice
1 clove crushed garlic
1 - 2 tablespoons fresh chopped parsley

Combine oil, juice, garlic and parsley in glass or china bowl. Cut squid into rings and quickly drop into boiling water for about 30 seconds, till it turns opaque (beware it's quick). Drain and toss in marinade. Refrigerate till next day. Serve as is, on a bed of salad greens with other salad vegetables or salsa to complement.

Marinated Squid with Lime and Coriander

2 squid tubes
Juice of 2 limes
2 tablespoons coriander

Marinade
½ cup cold pressed olive oil
2 cloves garlic crushed
Stalk lemon grass chopped
2 teaspoons palm sugar, organic honey or Date Mixture (see Miscellaneous)
1 chilli minced
Squeeze of lime juice extra

Combine marinade, then prepare squid. Cut squid tube down each side to separate into halves. Diagonally score inside of squid tube with a knife, first one way then the other to form a diamond pattern, being careful not to cut through the squid. Cut into large squares and place in flat glass or china dish if possible. Pour over marinade and leave for atleast ½ to 1 hour, turning from time to time to ensure all squid is covered. Have ready a hot griddle, barbecue or grill and toss quickly to cook until just opaque. Remember, overcooked seafood will be tough. Toss lime juice and coriander through cooked squid. Serve with a complementary salad or salsa.

Scallops in Basil Cream

250gms / ½lb scallops
2 limes juiced, lemon if limes unavailable
½ cup coconut cream
4 sprigs basil chopped
Sprinkle of Herbamare herbal salt and fresh ground black pepper
Lettuce cups

Place scallops in a bowl with lime juice and pepper. Cover and allow to marinate for atleast 4 hours, turning occasionally. (Can be left overnight). Stir in coconut cream and basil. Serve in lettuce cups on a platter, garnished with a small sprig of basil and lime slices, and add a complementary salad.

Egg 'Pizza'

4 organic free range eggs, lightly whisked with 2 tablespoons water
(over beating makes
    eggs tough)
¼ teaspoon Herbamare herbal seasoned salt
Fresh ground black pepper

Toppings
2 tomatoes sliced or sundried tomatoes
Anchovies drained (beware of oil they're in)
Chopped black olives (optional)
Slices of capsicum/pepper
Fresh pineapple chopped
Chopped basil or parsley
Any of your favourite toppings

**Have ready greased or oiled frypan on low to medium heat.
Gently pour in egg mixture and while it slowly sets from beneath
place desired toppings decoratively on top. When egg mixture
is set (all the runny bits have set) place fry pan (handle out of
course!) under moderate grill to gently set and brown on top. Cut
into wedges and serve with a complementary salad. This is also
delicious eaten cold for lunch or picnic. Serves 2.**

- To make more servings allow 2 eggs per person and a larger
  frypan if necessary.

Vegetarian Omelette

4 organic free range eggs
2 tablespoons water
6 - 8 mushrooms thinly sliced
2 shallots chopped
Dash Herbamare herbal seasoning salt
Fresh ground black pepper

Whisk eggs, water, herbal salt and pepper in a bowl without over beating. Add mushrooms and shallots. Have ready a moderately hot greased or oiled frypan and gently pour mixture into pan. Allow to set. When almost done place frypan under moderate grill to gently brown the top. Cut into wedges and serve with salad. Serves 2.

- For more servings allow 2 eggs per person and extra water, mushrooms and shallots.
- Add asparagus and shallots
- Add tomato and onion sliced, and chopped olives
- Add tomato sliced and anchovies
- Add tomato sliced, capsicum/pepper sliced and chopped shallots

Fresh Herbed Frittata

6 large organic free range eggs
2 cups fresh mixed herbs finely chopped, parsley, basil, chives,
coriander
2 tablespoons pecans, raw cashews, macadamia or pine nuts chopped
2 cloves garlic crushed
Dash Herbamare herb seasoned salt
Fresh ground black pepper

**Whisk eggs, herbal salt, pepper and garlic in a large bowl. Don't
over beat or the eggs will become tough. Stir in the nuts and
herbs. Pour into a moderately warm greased or oiled frypan
and allow to gently set. When almost done, place frypan
under moderate grill to finish setting the top and turn it a light
golden brown. Slice into wedges and eat warm served with a
complementary salad. Serves 4 – 6.**

- Also delicious served cold, especially as picnic food.

Egg Rolls

4 organic free range eggs
¼ cup water
Dash Herbamare herb seasoned salt

Fillings
- Fill with shredded lettuce, fresh sprouts and salsa of your choice
- Chop smoked salmon into strips with shredded lettuce, diced peach or mango and smear of home made mayonnaise
- Asparagus, strips of shallot, thin strips of tofu and smear of home made mayonnaise
- Rolled up with chopped tomatoes, fresh sprouts and herbs eg. chopped basil, thyme, parsley; and chopped black olives or anchovies

Whisk together eggs, water and herbed salt until just beaten. Over beating causes egg to be tough. Pour into moderately heated greased or oiled fry pan and allow to gently set. Spread with toppings of your choice, roll up and carefully lift from the pan. Serve with salad. Serves 2.

*This basic roll recipe is also in Lunchtime section with different fillings. As well as being great for picnic food or finger food, just make rolls thinner and cut into shorter lengths and they can be served as nibbles with drinks.

Stuffed Eggplant

2 eggplants halved lengthwise
2 onions finely chopped
3 medium tomatoes finely chopped
2 fresh cloves garlic crushed
½ cup each of fresh parsley and fresh basil chopped
Cold pressed olive oil
Sprinkle Herbamare herbal salt and fresh ground pepper
Mixed nuts finely crushed
Thin slices of butter/ghee or cold pressed olive oil

Combine all of above ingredients and heap on top of eggplant halves that have been brushed with oil. Sprinkle with nuts, top with butter/ghee or oil. Cook in a moderate oven for approximately an hour.

Salmon and Tomato Pasta

250gm / 8oz packet of rice pasta shells cooked according to instructions.
Large tin/canned pink salmon drained
400gms / ¾lb fresh tomatoes peeled and chopped
1 onion finely chopped
2 cloves garlic crushed
10 - 12 black olives halved and stoned
1 tablespoon capers rinsed under running water to remove white vinegar
4 tablespoons fresh basil shredded
2 tablespoons cold pressed olive oil
Freshly ground black pepper

Heat olive oil in pan and gently fry onion and garlic till soft. Add salmon, tomatoes, olives, capers and pepper, and cook gently for about 10 minutes. Drain cooked pasta shells and place into pasta bowls. Spoon over the sauce and garnish with the basil. Serve with complementary salad. Serves 4 to 6.

- In place of a tin/can salmon, add 2 cooked and flaked fresh salmon cutlets.

Pasta with Pesto

500gm / 1lb rice or rice/corn fettuccini or spaghetti
Pot of boiling salted water with a few drops of olive oil
1 quantity Pesto (see recipes below)

Boil fettuccini or spaghetti 10 to 12 minutes or until just cooked. Drain and toss the pesto through the fettuccini or spaghetti. Serve with complementary salad.

Italian Pesto

3 bunches fresh basil, (about 2 - 3 cups leaves)
1 tablespoon cold pressed olive oil
1 tablespoon chopped sundried tomatoes
2 cloves garlic crushed
2 tablespoons pine nuts
Fresh ground black pepper
¼ cup extra olive oil
*A minute sprinkle of parmesan cheese (optional)

Process basil, garlic, pine nuts and pepper in blender or food processor till smooth then slowly add the extra oil in a slow stream. Transfer mixture to a bowl until required.
*A sprinkle of parmesan cheese is for authentic flavour. I use about ½ teaspoon if I use it at all. Once pesto sits for a few hours the flavour of the parmesan permeates it so it isn't necessary to use large amounts of the cheese.

Cashew Pesto

2 cups fresh basil
¾ cup raw cashew pieces
1 tablespoon chopped sun-dried capsicum
2 cloves garlic crushed
1 cup cold pressed olive oil, sunflower, safflower or macadamia oil
*Sprinkle of parmesan cheese for flavour (optional - see above)

Gently brown cashews in a little olive oil and allow to cool. They brown quickly, be careful not to burn. Process all above ingredients in a blender or food processor, then sit aside to let flavours develop. Spread on crackers or rice cakes. Can be used as topping to rice / corn pasta.

Macadamia Pesto

½ cup macadamia nuts chopped
2 - 3 cups rocket/arugula chopped
2 tablespoon chopped sundried tomatoes
2 cloves garlic crushed
2 tablespoons of lemon juice
½ cup cold pressed olive oil
A dash of Herbamare herbal salt or organic sea salt
Fresh ground black pepper
*Sprinkle of parmesan cheese (optional - see above)

Blend all the ingredients but the oil, in a food processor. With the processor still running, slowly drizzle in the olive oil. Leave for a few hours till required. Spread on rice or corn cakes, or rice crackers. Toss through corn or rice pastas.

Pasta with Fresh Tomato Sauce

500gms / 1lb rice or rice/corn fettuccini or spaghetti cooked according to instructions
½ cup cold pressed olive oil
500gms / 1lb fresh ripe tomatoes finely chopped
1 onion finely chopped
2 cloves garlic crushed
6 black olives finely chopped
1 tablespoon capers rinsed under running water to remove white vinegar
1/3 cup fresh parsley finely chopped
½ teaspoon fresh oregano chopped, ¼ teaspoon dried if no fresh available

Combine all the above ingredients in a glass or china bowl and set aside in the refrigerator for some hours to allow flavours to develop. Return mixture to room temperature while spaghetti is cooking, then toss lightly through the hot spaghetti or fettuccini. Serve with a complementary salad. Serves 4.

Fresh Puttanesca and Pasta Salad

Cooked rice or rice/corn pasta eg spiral, penne pasta, fettuccine etc to serve 4 - 6 people
1 quantity of Tomato Herb Sauce (see Sauces)
3 anchovy fillets finely chopped
2 tablespoons capers rinsed under water to remove white vinegar
¼ cup chopped black olives

Stir the anchovies, capers and olives into the Herb Tomato Sauce and toss through the pasta or spoon over pasta in pasta bowls, and serve with a complementary salad.

Roasted Jacket Potatoes

4 organic, non-GMO potatoes, scrubbed and pricked with a fork
Butter/ghee or cold pressed oil with clove of crushed garlic (garlic optional but very
    nice)
Fresh chives finely chopped

Roll potatoes onto the rung in a moderate oven. Turn once or twice with tongs while cooking, about ¾ to 1 hour. Stab with a skewer to check. When ready to serve, take from the oven, cut a cross on top, being careful not to burn fingers, squeeze up and place a curl of butter/ghee or oil on top and sprinkle with chives.

- Serve up as an accompaniment to fish or game with an appropriate salad.
- Use in Hot Potato recipes in Lunch section.

Pakoras
(Savoury Fritters)

1 large eggplant sliced
1 onion separated into rings
Cauliflower florets
1 large red capsicum/pepper chopped into eight pieces
1 cup besan/chickpea flour
1 small red chilli finely chopped
½ teaspoon Herbamare herbal salt
½ teaspoon garam masala
2/3 cup water
Cold pressed olive oil or sunflower, safflower or macadamia

**Sift besan/chickpea flour into bowl with herbal salt, garam masala
and chopped chilli. Add water and beat into a smooth batter.
Coat vegetables in batter and quickly fry in hot oil, a few at a time
until crisp and golden brown. Drain well and serve while still
warm.**

Spiced Rice

2 cups brown long grain rice
3½ cups homemade organic chicken stock (see recipe Miscellaneous)
2 onions chopped
3 tablespoons cold pressed oil
8 peppercorns
5 cardamom pods crushed
2 cloves
1 stick cinnamon
A few saffron threads
½ teaspoon Herbamare herbal salt
½ cup natural sundried sultanas or raisins
1 cup slivered almonds, raw cashews or macadamia nuts

**In a large pan gently fry onions till soft. Add saffron and cook
another minute. Tip in rice and stir constantly to coat with
oil and turn golden. Pour in half the stock with peppercorns,
cardamom, cloves, cinnamon and herbal salt. Cover and simmer
till rice is tender, only putting in more stock as required. Add
sultanas or raisins and allow to sit until ready to serve, then add
almonds or other nuts, fluff rice with a fork, and tip into a large
bowl. Serves 8.**

Chicken Roll

750gms / 1½lb minced organic chicken
1/3 cup gluten-free breadcrumbs from rice bread or damper
2 tablespoons tomato sauce
1 egg
1 teaspoon dried mixed herbs
½ teaspoon Herbamare herb seasoned salt
Fresh ground black pepper

Filling
125gms /4 oz sulphur-free dried apricots chopped
¼ cup red capsicum/pepper finely chopped
½ cup cooked brown rice
1 small onion or 2 shallots finely chopped

Combine first group of ingredients in a bowl, making sure they are well mixed. Spread or roll meat out into a rectangular shape on a sheet of foil. Mix the filling ingredients together and spread evenly over meat. Using the foil, pick up one end and gently roll the meat so it folds like a Swiss roll. Then roll onto a greased tray and bake in a moderate oven for about 45 minutes. Remove from the oven and allow to cool. Chicken roll can be served hot but is even better left to go cold in the refrigerator and use as a cold cut of meat, accompanied with salad. Serves 6.

Nutloaf

3 slices rice bread or damper crumbled into breadcrumbs
2 cups almond milk or rice milk
150gms / 5oz ground hazelnuts
½ cup polenta
1 tablespoon arrowroot
2 eggs
2 tablespoons cold pressed oil
1 cup cooked brown rice
1 onion finely chopped
1 teaspoon kelp powder (optional)

**Mix all the ingredients together well and spoon into an oiled loaf
tin. Place tin in a pan of shallow water and cook in a moderate
oven till set, about 45 minutes. Serve hot or cold. Great for lunch
boxes.**

- Serve with Tomato Herb Sauce or another suitable sauce (see
  Sauces).
- Flavour loaf with 1 tablespoon home made curry powder for a
  change

Cabbage Rolls

10 cabbage leaves
2 cups cooked brown rice
1 cup minced organic chicken
1 cup macadamia or cashew nuts chopped
1 onion minced or finely chopped
½ cup celery finely diced
¼ teaspoon Herbamare herbal salt
1 level teaspoon mixed herbs
Fresh ground black pepper

**Quickly blanch cabbage leaves in boiling water to just soften then
remove. Combine remaining ingredients and fill each cabbage
leaf with heaped tablespoon of filling and roll into a parcel. Have
ready an oiled, ovenproof dish. Place rolls in. Cover and bake in
moderate oven, about 180°C / 350°F for 25 minutes. Serve with
Tomato Sauce.**

Tomato Sauce

4 cups tomatoes skinned and finely chopped
1 cup tomatoes pureed
2/3 cup mushrooms sliced
1 cup green capsicum/pepper finely chopped
1 cup celery finely sliced
1 tablespoon fresh basil leaves chopped
1 teaspoon ground cumin
Cold pressed olive oil
A sprinkle of Herbamare herbal salt
Fresh ground pepper

**Heat the oil in a pan and gently saute` mushrooms, celery and
capsicum/pepper. Add tomatoes and tomato puree, basil, cumin,
herbal salt and pepper, and simmer for about 10 minutes. Pour
over cabbage rolls and serve.**

Caponata

1 large eggplant cut into slices
4 large fresh ripe tomatoes chopped
1 red capsicum/pepper chopped
1 onion sliced
2 sticks celery sliced
1 tablespoon fresh thyme leaves
2 tablespoons capers rinsed under water to remove white vinegar
½ cup pitted green olives
3 tablespoons good cold pressed olive oil
2 tablespoons lemon juice
2 cloves garlic crushed
Dash of Herbamare herbal salt or organic sea salt
Grind of pepper (optional)
Lettuce leaves and fresh sprouts for serving

Lightly sprinkle both sides of eggplant slices with salt and leave to sit for about 30 minutes. Shake together the olive oil, lemon juice, crushed garlic, salt and pepper and set aside for flavours to develop. Rinse salt from eggplant and pat the slices dry. Fry quickly in a little olive oil in a fry pan till both sides are golden brown, then remove and cut into large cubes. Place in a bowl and lightly mix the dressing through and leave to marinate for atleast an hour. Gently toss with all remaining ingredients except the lettuce and sprouts. Serve in salad bowls on a bed of lettuce and the mixed sprouts.

Moroccan Eggplant Salad

2 large eggplant sliced about 1cm/½in thick
¼ cup cold pressed olive oil
4 large ripe organic tomatoes sliced into wedges
½ cup continental parsley leaves
½ cup pine nuts
2 cloves garlic crushed
1 chilli finely chopped
2 tablespoons lemon juice
2 tablespoons good cold pressed olive oil
½ teaspoon oregano chopped
¼ preserved lemon finely chopped
Dash of organic sea salt
Grind of pepper (optional)
Lettuce leaves to serve

**Brush both sides of eggplant slices with oil, lay on a baking tray
and cook in the oven at 180°C / 350°F until golden and crisp. In
a large bowl combine tomato wedges, parsley and pine nuts then
add cooked eggplant cut into pieces. Shake together remaining
ingredients in a screw top jar then gently toss through the salad.
Set aside at room temperature for atleast ½ to 1 hour, to allow
the flavours to blend. Serve in individual salad bowls on a bed of
lettuce leaves. Serves about 4.**

Pizza

1 pizza base (see Miscellaneous)

Toppings

Sun-dried Tomato and Olive
Tomato Herb Sauce (see Sauces)
1 cup sun-dried tomatoes
1 red capsicum/pepper cut into strips
1 onion sliced
½ cup black olives sliced
Clove garlic halved

Rub pizza base with halved garlic clove. Spread Tomato Herb Sauce over the pizza base. Top with onion slices, sun-dried tomatoes, capsicum/pepper and olives. Bake in a moderate oven about 180°C / 350°F for 20 to 30 minutes till base is cooked. Serve with an appropriate crisp lettuce salad of Italian flavour. Serves about 4.

Pesto and Tomato
1 cup fresh basil leaves roughly torn
2 tablespoons pine nuts
2 cloves garlic crushed
¼ cup good cold pressed olive oil
2 - 3 ripe tomatoes sliced
Dash of organic sea salt (optional)
Grind of fresh pepper (optional)

Process the basil leaves, pine nuts and crushed garlic in a blender till fine, then slowly drizzle in the olive oil. Spread this mixture over the pizza base and top with tomato slices. Sprinkle over sea salt very sparingly if desired, and a grind of fresh pepper. Bake in a moderately hot oven for 20 to 30 minutes till base is cooked. Serve with an appropriate salad.

- Top with any of your favourite toppings, fresh pineapple, onion, capsicum/pepper, anchovies, smoked fish, olives, dried tomatoes

SALADS IN A NUTSHELL

Salads can be made from any fruit, vegetable, nuts and herbs. We should try to eat as much of our food raw as possible. Because our bodies are made of live cells and enzymes so our bodies should be fed live food, as fresh and as natural (free of genetic engineering, pesticides, herbicides and artificial fertilizer) as we can acquire. Listed below are more suggestions for delicious, invigorating and energizing salads.

- Use as many salad greens as possible, these include all the different types of lettuce, spinach and silver beet, rocket/arugula, mizuna, endive, chicory and mustards
- Add sundried tomatoes, especially if marinated in olive oil
- Use lots of sprouts alfalfa, fenugreek, mung bean, onion and radish
- Add edible flower petals such as calendula, nasturtium or rose
- Add chopped leaves of nasturtium and dandelion
- Use lots of grated fresh coconut, rich in many essential vitamins, minerals and oils
- Add raw nuts and seeds wherever possible. Nuts and greens form a complete protein
- Seeds – sunflower, pumpkin/pepita, fennel, cumin, dill, caraway, celery or poppy
- Use lots of herbs, for flavor as well as natural medicines.
- Add fresh raw snow peas/mange tout, ordinary peas, beans sliced, grated turnip or swede/rutabaga, always grated carrot.
- Add lots of raw beetroot for nourishment of the nervous system and brain, blood and bone development, hormones and to detoxify the liver
- Dried seaweed – crumbled or soaked and cut into shreds

From the cold pressed oils in the dressings we obtain some of our essential fatty acids required by the body, the lemon juice is rich in phosphorus, sodium (for the elimination of wastes from our body) and vitamin C, and any herbs and garlic we add are our medicine. So, as well as adding extra zing to our food, they give added nutritional value.

Rich Red Salad

2 sliced tomatoes
1 cup shredded beetroot
1 cup shredded cabbage
1 small finely chopped onion
1 cup shredded carrot
Green lettuce leaves
Fresh sprouts
Home made mayonnaise (see Dressings)

**Toss beetroot, cabbage, onion and carrot lightly. Serve on bed of
lettuce leaves and fresh sprouts, decorated with tomato slices and
a good dollop of mayonnaise.**

Vegetable Salad

1 cup shredded beetroot
1 cup diced celery
1 small cucumber diced
1 cup sliced radishes
½ cup shredded cabbage
½ cup finely chopped shallots
Lettuce leaves and fresh sprouts to serve
Home made mayonnaise (see Dressings)

**Toss first five ingredients lightly. Serve on a bed of lettuce and
sprouts with a good dollop of mayonnaise on top.**

Green and Gold Salad

1 cup shredded cabbage
1 cup grated raw turnip
1 cup chopped green beans
½ cup finely chopped shallots
Lettuce leaves and fresh sprouts for serving
Homemade mayonnaise (see Dressings) to which chives has been added

Toss first four ingredients lightly together. Serve on a bed of lettuce and sprouts with a good dollop of mayonnaise on top.

• Add Blood Orange Mayonnaise for a wonderful flavour.

Sweet and Sour Salad

1 small lettuce torn into pieces
2 carrots coarsely grated
1 tart apple eg Granny Smith, coarsely grated
2 sticks celery sliced
4-5 radishes thinly sliced
1 small onion sliced
1 sprig fresh parsley chopped
Wholegrain Mustard Dressing, with a little fresh pineapple juice or orange juice added
Raw nuts roughly chopped - macadamias, pecans, almonds, pine nuts; or seeds -
    sunflower seeds, pepitas (pumpkin seeds) etc

In a large bowl combine the lettuce, carrots, apple, celery, radishes, onion and parsley and lightly toss. Just before serving, sprinkle through the chopped nuts and/or seeds and toss through the dressing.

A Bowl of Salad

4 - 6 cups mixed lettuce leaves torn into pieces
½ bunch of rocket/arugula (optional)
12 cherry tomatoes, halved or 3 medium tomatoes in wedges
1 Spanish onion sliced or shallots in strips
1 Lebanese cucumber sliced
½ cup sprouts
1 tablespoon torn basil leaves or 1 teaspoon fresh thyme leaves
2 sprigs of parsley chopped
Salad dressing (see Dressings)

In a large bowl, lightly toss all above ingredients, except dressing. Just before serving toss through salad dressing and serve.

Mango with Smoked Salmon Salad

6 cups mixed lettuce leaves torn into pieces
1 bunch rocket/arugula torn into pieces
200gms / 6oz smoked salmon cut into strips
2 mangoes peeled and cubed
1 avocado cubed
1 medium Spanish onion sliced or shallots chopped
1 Lebanese cucumber cubed
Honey Mustard Dressing or similar appropriate dressing (see Dressings)

In a large bowl, lightly toss all of above ingredients except the dressing. Just before serving, toss through honey mustard or similar dressing. Serves 4 - 6.

Smoked Salmon and Pear Salad

4 cups mixed lettuce leaves torn into pieces
1 bunch rocket/arugula
200gms / 6oz smoked salmon cut into strips
2 pears peeled, cored and cubed
1 Spanish onion sliced
1 red capsicum/pepper cut in strips
1 avocado cubed
Capers (optional - but wash in strainer to remove as much vinegar as possible)
Honey Mustard Dressing or similar dressing (see Dressings)

In a bowl, lightly toss together all the ingredients except the dressing. Just before serving, toss through honey mustard dressing. Serves 4 - 6.

Potato / Sweet Potato Salad

500gms / 1lb red sweet potato, peeled and diced, or normal GM-free potatoes
1 salad onion or 3 shallots and tops finely chopped
2 good sprigs of mint finely chopped
Juice of a lemon

Cook sweet potato in boiling salted water until just tender. Drain and add onion, mint and lemon juice. Gently toss, tip into bowl and refrigerate till required.

Colourful Coleslaw

2 cups red cabbage, finely shredded
2 cups white cabbage, finely shredded
1 cup grated carrot
1 stalk celery finely sliced
½ green or yellow capsicum/pepper finely chopped
1 small onion or shallots finely chopped
½ teaspoon celery seeds
1 teaspoon dill seeds
1 teaspoon caraway seeds
Homemade mayonnaise with cayenne added (see Mayonnaises)

Combine all the salad ingredients in a large bowl and set aside till required. A few minutes before serving toss through the mayonnaise.

Vegetable Coleslaw

2 cups cabbage, finely shredded
1 cup finely shredded silver beet or spinach
1 cup grated carrot
½ cup grated apple
½ cup grated turnip
3 radishes sliced
1 small onion, finely diced
1 stalk celery finely sliced
Homemade mayonnaise (see recipe in Mayonnaises)

Combine all the salad vegetables in a large bowl, and set aside till required. A few minutes before serving, lightly toss through the mayonnaise.

- Try Blood Orange Mayonnaise
- Add chopped chives or seeds eg fennel, dill, caraway to the mayonnaise

Red Slaw

6 apples, grated
2 small beetroot, grated
1 grated carrot
½ stalk of celery finely sliced
Fresh orange juice
Sprig of fresh mint, finely chopped
Cinnamon, nutmeg

Pour orange juice over grated apple. Add beetroot, carrot, celery and chopped mint. Sprinkle with a light dusting of cinnamon and nutmeg. Dressing not required for this slaw as the orange juice, as well as preventing apple discolouring, also serves as the dressing.

Pineapple Coleslaw

2 cups cabbage shredded
1 cup chopped fresh pineapple
1 cup grated carrot
1 Spanish onion, finely chopped
4 radishes, thinly sliced
2 good sprigs of mint or parsley, finely chopped
Home made mayonnaise (see Dressings)

Combine all of the ingredients but the mayonnaise, in a bowl. A few minutes before serving lightly toss through the mayonnaise.

Fruit and Nut Coleslaw

4 cups cabbage finely shredded
2 cups fresh pineapple finely chopped
1 cup grated carrot
2 tablespoons fresh chopped chives
½ cup pine nuts or chopped macadamia nuts
1/3 cup lime or lemon juice
1/3 cup fresh orange juice
½ cup cold pressed oil eg. olive, macadamia, sunflower, safflower or mixture
1 teaspoon Dijon mustard

Place shredded cabbage, pineapple, carrot, pine nuts or chopped macadamias and chives into serving bowl. Combine juice, oil and mustard in a screw top jar and shake till well mixed. Gently toss dressing through the coleslaw, cover and refrigerate until required.

Cabbage and Date Coleslaw

4 cups cabbage shredded
8 dates finely chopped
1 tart apple diced (sprinkled with lemon, lime or orange juice)
1 carrot grated
1 onion finely chopped
Spicy Coleslaw Dressing - this is not hot spicy (see Dressings)

In a large bowl, combine the cabbage, dates, apple, carrot and onion. Toss through the Spicy Coleslaw Dressing and leave to marinate for about an hour before serving.

- Refreshing alternative, replace apple with chopped pineapple and shavings of fresh coconut.
- Add ½ a red capsicum/pepper diced for extra color, nutrition and flavor.

Sweet Corn and Cabbage Slaw

2 fresh cobs of corn, kernels sliced from the cob
2 cups shredded fresh cabbage
1 carrot grated
1 red capsicum/pepper finely diced
1 small onion finely diced
½ cup homemade mayonnaise
1 tablespoon chopped mint
1 tablespoon chopped chives
Lemon or lime juice to taste

Mix together mayonnaise, mint, chives and lemon/lime juice and set aside till required. Combine the remaining ingredients in a large bowl and gently toss through the mayonnaise. Refrigerate till ready to serve.

Carrot and Apricot Salad

2 carrots shredded
8 - 10 apricots diced (or dried apricots that have been soaked in filtered water)
2 stalks celery large diced
3 shallots and green tops sliced
2 tablespoons chopped parsley
Lemon or lime juice or light dressing (see Dressings)
Lettuce leaves and fresh sprouts

Combine all the salad ingredients in a bowl and squeeze fresh lemon or lime juice over. Lightly toss and serve on a bed of lettuce and sprouts.

Carrot and Coconut Salad

2 cups carrot grated
½ cup grated fresh coconut
½ cup currants
¼ cup lemon juice or lime juice

Toss all the above ingredients together and refrigerate for at least an hour, to allow the flavours to develop and currants to plump.

Citrus Salad

6 oranges, peeled and thinly sliced
2 large salad onions, thinly sliced
½ cup black olives
1 clove of crushed garlic
French Dressing (see dressings)

Layer the orange slices and onion rings on a platter, and decorate with olives. Add crushed garlic to dressing and spoon over the salad just before serving. Serves 4.

Mango and Anchovy Rice Salad

1 mignonette lettuce, leaves separated
Fresh sprouts
3 cups cooked brown rice
1 mango, diced
6 - 8 anchovies in oil, drained and halved
3 shallots sliced
2 avocadoes, sliced
1/3 cup of French dressing (see Dressings)
1 clove of crushed garlic, added to dressing

Line a platter with lettuce leaves and fresh sprouts. Gently toss the cooked rice, mango, onion, anchovies and dressing, and heap onto lettuce and sprout lined platter. Decorate with avocado slices. Serves about 4.

Mango and Avocado Salad

2 avocadoes, peeled, quartered, then sliced crosswise
2 mangoes, peeled, sliced
½ cup pecans
6 - 8 anchovy fillets, drained
1 mignonette lettuce, torn into pieces
French dressing (see Dressings)

**Gently toss the above ingredients, except dressing, lightly
together. When ready to serve, toss with dressing. Serves 6.**

Country Garden Salad

4 - 6 cups salad greens, torn into pieces and mixed sprouts
1 punnet cherry tomatoes
100gms / 4oz snow peas/mange tout, halved
1 salad onion thinly sliced
6 mushrooms thinly sliced
Sprigs of dill or parsley
French Dressing (see Dressings)

**Toss all the salad and herb ingredients together in a large bowl,
and just before serving, toss with the dressing. Serves 4.**

Fresh Beetroot Salad

4 medium beetroot
4 oranges
½ cup pecans roughly broken
2 green shallots chopped
Ginger Dressing (see Dressings)

**Coarsely grate or finely shred beetroot. Peel oranges thickly and
cut into segments. Arrange orange segments and beetroot on a
plate. Top with pecans and chopped shallots. Pour over Ginger
Dressing and serve. Serves 6.**

Good Lunchtime Salad

6 cups of salad greens, torn into pieces
1 cup shredded carrot
1 cup pecans
3 tablespoons chopped parsley
2 tablespoons sunflower seeds
2 tablespoons pine nuts
2 tomatoes cut into thin wedges
1 small avocado, diced
2 hard boiled eggs, quartered (optional)
French Dressing (see Dressings)
Fresh alfalfa sprouts for garnish

Arrange the salad greens on a platter or in a bowl. In a large bowl combine the remaining ingredients, except the dressing. Just before serving, gently toss through the dressing and heap onto the platter and garnish with mixed sprouts. Serves about 4 - 6.

Tropical Sunshine Salad

½ fresh pineapple cubed
2 carrots grated coarsely
½ cup grated fresh coconut
½ green capsicum/pepper chopped
2 sticks celery thinly sliced
2 cups lettuce greens torn into pieces
½ cup sultanas
½ teaspoon celery seeds
Mayonnaise with mustard added or French Dressing (see Mayonnaises and Dressings)
Fresh mixed sprouts

Combine all the ingredients, but the dressing, in a bowl. Just before serving toss lightly with the dressing or serve the dressing on side. Garnish with mixed sprouts.

Waldorf Salad

Mixed salad greens and sprouts e.g. alfalfa, radish, onion, fenugreek
1 cup of diced apple
1 cup diced celery
½ cup walnuts or pecans
½ cup fresh grated coconut
½ cup homemade mayonnaise (see Mayonnaises)
Sprigs of mint

**Toss together the apple, celery, walnuts, coconut and mayonnaise.
Serve heaped on a bed of salad greens and sprouts, garnished with
sprigs of mint.**

Tomato and Herb Salad

8 tomatoes, sliced
4 tablespoons parsley, chopped
2 tablespoons basil, chopped
2 tablespoons thyme, chopped
4 spring onions, finely chopped
1 crushed clove of garlic
6 tablespoons cold pressed olive oil
3 tablespoons lemon juice
1 teaspoon organic honey (optional)
Fresh ground pepper

**Mix all the ingredients, except the tomatoes, together to make
the dressing. Arrange layers of tomatoes on a platter with herbed
dressing between each layer. Refrigerate till ready to serve. Serves
4 - 6.**

Cauliflower Salad

½ small head of cauliflower broken into small florets
1 avocado in large dice
½ cup red capsicum/pepper, chopped
½ cup celery, chopped
1 small onion or shallots, sliced
2 tablespoons fresh basil, chopped
2 tablespoons fresh parsley, chopped
½ cup of homemade mayonnaise with a good squeeze lemon juice
added

**Toss all lightly together and refrigerate until required. This salad
is a good accompaniment to seafood. Serves 4.**

Potato Salad with Salmon Dressing

1 kg / 2lb small new organic potatoes
4 green shallots, sliced
6 hard boiled organic eggs, quartered
1 tablespoon capers (wash under running water to remove vinegar)
Salmon Dressing (see Dressings)

**Boil or steam potatoes until tender. Drain and place in a salad
bowl. Add shallots, eggs and capers. Pour over the dressing and
toss lightly. Can be served hot or cold. Serves 6.**

Salmon Bean Salad

Large tin/can of pink salmon, flaked
4 - 6 cups salad greens, torn into pieces and mixed sprouts
500gms / 1lb shelled raw broad beans
1 small salad onion, thinly sliced
6 tablespoons cold pressed olive oil
3 tablespoons lemon juice
Black olives, stoned
1 tablespoon parsley, chopped
1 tablespoon oregano or marjoram, chopped
Fresh ground black pepper

Make a dressing from the olive oil and lemon juice. In a large bowl combine all the remaining ingredients, except lettuce greens and sprouts, and toss lightly with the dressing. Arrange lettuce greens and sprouts on a platter and heap the bean salad in the middle and serve. Serves 4 - 6.

* In place of tinned/canned salmon use 3 cooked, flaked, fresh salmon cutlets.

Snow pea/Mange Tout Salad

250gms / ½lb snow peas/mange tout with ends trimmed
2 shallots sliced
2 heaped tablespoons chervil (chopped chives if chervil unavailable)
2 tablespoons raw small cashew nut pieces or pine nuts
Homemade French dressing
Fresh ground pepper

Toss the above ingredients together and marinate till required (atleast 1 hour). Garnish with a sprig of parsley.

Tomato, Celery and Zucchini Salad

3 medium tomatoes cut into wedges
1 stalk celery, cut into 4cm/1½in strips
1 medium zucchini, sliced
10 kalamata olives
150gms / 5oz organic *tofu, cubed (can be purchased flavored with chives etc)
2 - 3 tablespoons fresh basil, chopped
Basic dressing

Place all in a bowl, finishing with the dressing. Refrigerate for an hour or two before required. Serves 4.
* Tofu (soy product) is a special treat. Watch for any reactions.

Salmon Salad with a Touch of Tarragon

6 cups mixed salad greens
3 Atlantic salmon steaks cooked and flaked
2 large tomatoes chopped into wedges
250gms / ½lb fresh green beans chopped in 4cm / 1½ pieces
1 small cucumber sliced
¼ cup tarragon leaves chopped
2 tablespoons snipped chives
Homemade mayonnaise

Add tarragon leaves and chives to the mayonnaise and sit aside. Combine the remaining ingredients on a serving platter or in individual salad bowls. Dribble over the mayonnaise and serve. Serves 4.

- Salmon steaks can be substituted with 500gms / 1lb cooked organic chicken.
- In place of salmon steaks use a large tin/can of pink salmon.

Fennel and Dried Tomato Salad

1 small fennel bulb, sliced into thin rounds
½ cup dried tomatoes chopped
1 tablespoon capers (rinse well with water to remove white vinegar)
2 cups mixed lettuce leaves including rocket/arugula, endive and spinach
2 tablespoon pine nuts (optional)
Simple Lemon Mustard Dressing (see Dressings)

Gently toss all ingredients together in a bowl, lastly pouring on the dressing. Serve as a side salad with egg dishes or fish. This salad can be eaten as a meal on its own because pine nuts and greens make a complete protein.

Grape and Walnut Salad

4 cups mixture of lettuce leaves or rocket/arugula leaves, butter lettuce and radicchio
1 cup of green grapes
½ cup walnut halves
1 tablespoon chopped fresh chives
Wholegrain Mustard Dressing (see Dressings)

Make the dressing and set aside to allow the flavours to develop. In a large salad bowl toss together the lettuce leaves, grapes, chives and walnut halves. Just before serving, gently toss the dressing through.

Beetroot Salad

3 small fresh beetroot grated or julienned into straws
2 tablespoons shallots finely chopped
1 small sprig fresh thyme
3 tablespoons cold pressed olive oil, or mix of olive and macadamia
oil
2 tablespoons lemon or lime juice
Dash of Herbamare herbal salt
A grind of pepper (optional)

In a bowl, combine the beetroot, shallots and the thyme leaves that have been stripped from their stems. Pour the oil, juice, salt and pepper into a jar. Place on lid and shake. Lightly toss this dressing through the salad and set aside a while till ready to serve, to allow the flavours to develop. Serve at table with other salads.

- In place of lemon or lime juice, add orange juice and a dash of fresh ground allspice for an exotic flavour.
- Add some pine nuts or roughly chopped macadamia nuts for extra protein and essential nutrients.

Tomato Salad

3 large ripe tomatoes cut in wedges
1 cup mixed salad greens - mixed lettuce leaves, rocket/arugula, mizuna, baby spinach
1 avocado quartered and sliced
½ red capsicum/pepper cut into strips
½ cup grated carrot
½ cup celery
½ cup thinly sliced fennel
¼ - ½ cup sunflower seeds or pine nuts
2 tablespoons chopped fresh parsley
Good cold pressed olive oil or macadamia nut oil
2 teaspoons apricot kernel oil
½ lemon juiced

In a large salad bowl, combine all of the fruits and vegetables. Just before serving pour over about 2 tablespoons of olive oil and a teaspoon or two of apricot kernel oil, squeeze over the lemon juice and gently toss through.

- For a change of flavour, remove parsley and add torn fresh basil leaves
- To add Greek touch, throw in some olives
- Toss through chopped anchovy fillets
- Add chopped onion or shallots

Pear Salad

2 large pears cored and sliced
2 avocadoes sliced
Cucumber slices
Lettuce leaves torn into pieces
2 tablespoons broken pecan nuts
1 tablespoon chopped chives
Coconut Dressing (see Dressings)

Place torn lettuce leaves on a serving platter. Arrange the pear, avocado and cucumber slices on top. Sprinkle around the pecans then garnish with the chives. Just before serving, drizzle over the dressing. Serves about 4.

• Rather than chives as a garnish, for something different use poppy or fennel seeds

Pear and Turnip Salad

1 head lettuce (butter lettuce, oak leaf lettuce etc) torn into bite-size pieces
4 pears in large cubes (sprinkled with lemon, lime or orange juice)
1 fresh turnip coarsely grated
2 small onions sliced
1 tablespoon chopped fresh mint
1/3 cup walnut pieces
Light oil and lemon juice dressing (see Dressings) or try a mayonnaise

In a large bowl, combine the lettuce, pears, grated turnip, onion and mint. When ready to serve. sprinkle the nuts over and lightly toss through the dressing.

Pear and Baby Spinach Salad

3 ripe pears cored, diced and coated in a little lemon juice
250gms / 8oz fresh baby spinach leaves or fresh silverbeet leaves torn
into pieces
1 red capsicum/pepper cut into strips
1 shallot finely sliced, green top included
Juice of half lemon
3 tablespoons walnut oil, or a mixture of cold pressed apricot kernel
and avocado oil
1 teaspoon homemade mustard (see Miscellaneous)
Sprinkle of Herbamare herbal salt
Fresh ground black pepper

**Lightly toss pears, spinach, capsicum/pepper and shallot in a
serving bowl. In a glass jar shake oil, lemon juice, Herbamare salt
and pepper, and pour over salad just before serving. Garnish with
a few walnuts and small sprig of parsley.**

Tropical Delight

2 avocadoes sliced
2 mangoes peeled and sliced
2 pineapple slices cut into pieces
1 carrot julienned into straws
1 red capsicum/pepper julienned into straws
1 stalk of celery julienned into straws
8 thin slices of cucumber
Mignonette lettuce leaves or similar lettuce
1 tablespoon parsley finely chopped to garnish
Pineapple Dressing (see Dressings)

Spread lettuce leaves on a platter and decoratively arrange fruit and vegetables on top, lastly the cucumber rounds in the centre. Sprinkle chopped parsley over the fruits. Just before serving drizzle over the Pineapple Dressing. Serves 4 - 6.

- This salad can be served with pieces of raw marinated fish or cold cooked fish added to make a main dish
- Add macadamia nuts or mixture of nuts to this salad. In combination with the lettuce and parsley the nuts make the salad a main meal.

Asparagus and Blood Orange Salad

1 bunch fresh asparagus, chopped into 3cm / 1½in lengths
1 blood orange, peeled but retaining some pith, segmented and each
segment halved
1 tablespoon mint or chives finely chopped
Lettuce leaves
Blood Orange Mayonnaise (see Mayonnaises and Dressings)

**In a bowl, toss together the asparagus, blood orange pieces and
mint. Serve on a platter lined with lettuce leaves, and drizzle with
Blood Orange Dressing. Offer at table with other salad selections.**

- Replace blood orange with ruby red grapefruit for a refreshing
  salad that is also a digestive aid.
- Asparagus is a highly nutritious vegetable if it hasn't been cooked

Rice Salad

2 cups cooked brown rice
1 cup fresh raw shelled peas
Small fresh cob of corn kernels (trimmed from the cob with a sharp
knife)
½ red capsicum/pepper finely chopped
1 small red onion finely chopped
1 tablespoon fresh coriander leaves
1 teaspoon fennel seeds
1 teaspoon ground cumin
Nut Dressing (see Dressings)

**First, mix together the rice, fennel seeds and ground cumin. Toss
through the remaining ingredients, lastly the dressing. Set aside
till ready to serve, to allow the flavours to develop.**

- In place of Nut Dressing toss through Pineapple Dressing or
  Coconut Dressing
- Add a chopped mango, peaches, fresh pineapple pieces or citrus
  for a different flavour.

Thai Rice Salad

2 cups cooked brown rice
1 red capsicum/pepper finely sliced
1 avocado cubed
2 bananas cubed and sprinkled with orange juice
1 small cucumber diced
2 tablespoons raisins
2 tablespoons cashews
1 orange juiced (use some of juice to sprinkle on apple)
Sprig of coriander
Thai Dressing (see Dressings) or a dressing of choice

While brown rice cooks, soak raisins in orange juice to plump. In a large bowl toss together the cold rice, capsicum/pepper, cucumber, raisins and cashews, then gently mix in the avocado, banana and the dressing. Garnish with sprig of coriander and chill till ready to serve. Serves 4.

Asparagus, Peas and Corn Salad

½ bunch asparagus spears chopped into 2cm pieces
10 fresh snow peas/mange tout or sugar snap peas sliced diagonally
1 small cob fresh corn, the kernels sliced from its cob
½ red capsicum/pepper diced
Lettuce leaves
Citrus flavoured mayonnaise of your choice
1 tablespoon chopped fresh chives

Mix the chives into the mayonnaise and set aside till required. Combine the asparagus, snow peas, corn and capsicum/pepper and serve on lettuce leaves. Drizzle over the mayonnaise.

- Try a spicy mayonnaise in place of a citrus mayonnaise.
- In place of asparagus, add bean sprouts, chopped mint and coriander.

Green Salad with Lemon or Lime Coconut Dressing

250gms / ½lb fresh crisp green beans sliced into 5cm / 2in lengths
1 green capsicum/pepper julienned into 5cm / 2in lengths
2 small cucumbers julienned into 5cm / 2in lengths
6 shallots julienned into 5cm / 2in lengths
1 cup fresh shredded coconut
½ cup coconut cream
¼ cup lemon or lime juice
2 cloves garlic crushed
2 tablespoons freshly chopped mint

To make the dressing, blend the coconut cream, lemon or lime juice, garlic and mint and set aside to allow the flavours to develop. In a salad bowl, combine beans, capsicum/pepper, cucumbers and shallots. On a large salad platter or individual plates, place a bed of shredded coconut, top with the vegetables then spoon over the dressing.

Fay's Eggplant Salad

1 eggplant sliced and brushed with cold pressed olive oil
1 small red capsicum/pepper diced*
2 medium ripe tomatoes diced
1 clove garlic crushed*
A little finely diced chilli if desired
Dash organic sea salt or Herbamare herbal salt
A little good quality cold pressed olive oil

Grill the eggplant slices on both sides then remove the skin and cube. In a bowl, combine the eggplant, capsicum/red pepper, tomatoes, garlic and chilli. Sprinkle with a dash of organic sea salt or Herbamare and lightly toss with olive oil to taste.

*Fay blisters and peels the capsicum/pepper and crushes the garlic with salt, but for maximum nutrition we prefer not to do this.

SALSAS

Pineapple Coconut Salsa

1½ cups of finely chopped fresh pineapple
½ bunch fresh coriander, chopped
½ cup shredded or grated fresh coconut
1 teaspoon grated ginger
1 tablespoon fresh lime juice
Fresh ground black pepper to taste

Mix all ingredients together and chill until required. Serve with eggs, seafood, organic chicken or duck. This is also a suitable topping for tacos or tortillas.

Apple Salsa

1 Granny Smith apple, peeled, cored and finely chopped
2 shallots or 1 Spanish onion finely chopped
1 clove crushed garlic
½ to 1 teaspoon chopped chilli (optional)
1 tablespoon chopped coriander
Juice of 1 lime, ½ teaspoon grated zest

Mix all ingredients together in bowl and leave till required. Serve with fish, especially good with cooked trout and Atlantic salmon fillets or organic chicken. Serves approximately 4.

Garden Salsa

2 ripe tomatoes, finely chopped
1 Lebanese cucumber finely chopped
1 red capsicum/pepper finely chopped
1 Spanish onion chopped
2 teaspoons finely chopped basil
2 tablespoons lemon juice

Combine all the ingredients in a bowl until required. Serve with omelette, fish fillets or cooked slices of eggplant. Serves approximately 4.

• Add a dash of Tabasco Sauce to give the salsa a zing.

Kiwi Salsa

3 kiwi fruit, peeled and finely chopped
1 teaspoon honey (optional)
1 shallot finely sliced
1 bunch chopped fresh mint
2 tablespoons lemon or lime juice

Combine above ingredients in a bowl and set aside until required. This is a suitable accompaniment to fish and other sea foods.

Mango Salsa

2 mangoes peeled and finely diced
1 small Spanish onion or shallots chopped finely
1 Lebanese cucumber finely diced
1/3 cup grated fresh coconut
2 tablespoons chopped coriander
½ teaspoon chopped chilli (optional)
4 tablespoons cold pressed olive oil
2 tablespoons lime juice or lemon juice
Fresh ground black pepper

Combine all but olive oil, lime juice and pepper in a bowl. Pour olive oil, juice and pepper into a jar and shake till well combined. Pour over salsa and set aside till required. Serve with fish, seafood, omelette or topping with shredded lettuce for tortillas. Serves 4.

Hot Peach Salsa

3 large ripe peaches, diced
1 red capsicum/pepper finely diced
1 Spanish onion finely diced
3 tablespoons fresh coriander chopped
3 tablespoons chopped fresh parsley
½ teaspoon chilli finely chopped
1 tablespoon organic honey (optional)
1 crushed clove of garlic
2 tablespoons lime juice or 1 of lime and 1 of orange (and omit the honey)
4 tablespoons cold pressed olive oil

Combine the first six salsa ingredients in a bowl. Shake together the honey, oil and lime juice or lime/orange juice in a jar and pour over the salsa. Serve with fish, rice or as a topping with shredded lettuce on tortillas. Serves approximately 6.

Avocado Salsa

2 avocadoes diced
2 tomatoes diced
1 chili seeded and minced (optional)
3 tablespoons fresh coriander, chopped
¼ teaspoon ground cumin
A sprinkle of Herbamare herbal salt
4 tablespoons cold pressed olive oil
2 tablespoons lime juice

Combine the first four salsa ingredients in a bowl. Shake together the oil, cumin, herbal salt and juice in a jar and pour over salsa. Set aside till required. Serves 4.

Avocado & Kiwifruit Salsa

1 large avocado, diced
2 kiwifruit peeled and finely diced
1 shallot finely sliced
1 tablespoon lime or lemon juice
1 tablespoon fresh chives finely chopped
½ teaspoon minced chili (optional)
Fresh ground black pepper

Gently toss all the above ingredients together in a bowl, cover and refrigerate till required. A great accompaniment to fish or an egg dish.

Paw paw/Papaya and Kiwifruit Salsa

3 kiwifruit peeled and diced
¼ paw paw/papaya peeled and finely diced
1 clove of garlic crushed
1 tablespoon fresh chives chopped
1 tablespoon lime or lemon juice

Gently toss the above ingredients in a bowl and set aside in refrigerator till required. A great accompaniment with fish, seafood or egg dish.

Capsicum/Pepper Salsa

½ red capsicum/pepper finely chopped
½ green capsicum/pepper finely chopped
6 shallots finely sliced (green tops also)
1 small red onion finely chopped
1 small red chilli seeded and chopped (optional)
2 tablespoons fresh mint chopped
¼ cup lime juice

Combine all ingredients in a bowl, and set aside till ready to serve. A great accompaniment to fish or egg dishes, in tacos or as a topping on shredded lettuce for tortillas. Serves 4.

Mango and Ginger Salsa

2 large ripe mangoes peeled and diced
2 tablespoons shallots and green tops chopped
1 teaspoon fresh ginger grated
1 chilli finely chopped (optional)
2 tablespoons chopped mint leaves
4 tablespoons chopped fresh coriander
1 tablespoon fresh lemon or lime juice

Combine all ingredients in a bowl and set aside till required. Makes about 2 cups. Serve with fish or egg dish, or serve with other salads.

• In place of mangoes, 4 delicious, ripe, organic yellow peaches make a wonderful salsa.

Tomato Basil Salsa

4 egg tomatoes finely diced
1 tablespoon capers well rinsed to remove white vinegar
1 tablespoon basil finely chopped
¼ cup good cold pressed olive oil
Grind of pepper (optional)
Lemon or lime juice

Combine diced tomatoes, basil and capers, and drizzle with olive oil. Flavour with lemon or lime juice and fresh pepper to taste. Set aside till required.

Tuscany Salsa

2 ripe tomatoes finely diced
1 small salad onion finely diced
1 tablespoon finely diced olives
1 tablespoon finely chopped basil

Combine all ingredients in a bowl and refrigerate till required.

Salsa Mexicana

2 ripe tomatoes finely diced
½ red capsicum/pepper finely diced
1 cob of fresh corn - slice kernels from the cob with a sharp knife
1 stick celery finely diced
1 small red onion finely diced
1 teaspoon Mexican tarragon, finely chopped or coriander or parsley
2 tablespoons cold pressed olive oil
1 clove garlic crushed
1 teaspoon honey (optional)
Dash chilli powder

In a jar, shake together the oil, garlic, honey and dash of chilli powder. Combine the remaining salsa ingredients in a bowl and pour over the dressing. Set aside until ready to serve. An accompaniment for egg dishes or fish and seafood, and as a topping with shredded lettuce for tortillas or tacos (see Lunch recipes).

Hot Pineapple Salsa

3 cups finely chopped pineapple
1 small red onion finely diced
2 tablespoons fresh chopped coriander
1 small red chilli finely diced
2 tablespoons fresh lime juice
1 teaspoon grated lime rind

Combine all the ingredients, lightly tossing through the lime juice. Set aside till ready to serve. This salsa is a good accompaniment for fish and other sea foods. Serves 4.

- Serve in lettuce cups as a salad.
- Toss some macadamia nut pieces through.
- Use with shredded lettuce as a filling for egg rolls, tacos and tortillas.

MAYONNAISE, DRESSINGS & SAUCES

The finishing touch to a good salad - a mayonnaise
or dressing can make a very boring salad
into a gourmet's delight.

Basic Dressing

4 tablespoons cold pressed olive oil and/or macadamia nut, safflower,
sunflower oil
4 tablespoons lemon or lime juice
Fresh ground pepper (optional)

Pour into sealed jar and shake. Set aside till required.

• To this can be added herbs such as thyme, chopped chives,
  parsley, mint etc, seeds such as dill, coriander, ground fenugreek,
  mustard seed or ½ - to 1 teaspoon home made seeded mustard or
  some spices.

Honey Mustard Dressing

2 tablespoons cold pressed olive oil
2 tablespoons lime or lemon juice
1 teaspoon of lime or lemon zest (optional)
2 teaspoons grain mustard
2 teaspoons organic honey or replace with Date Sweetener (See
Miscellaneous)

Whisk all above ingredients and leave till required.

Ginger Dressing

¼ cup cold pressed olive oil
1 teaspoon organic honey, organic maple syrup or Date Sweetener
(see Miscellaneous)
¼ cup orange juice
Juice of 2 limes
1/2 teaspoon grated lime zest
1 teaspoon grated ginger

Whisk all ingredients together and stand aside till required.

French Dressing

2/3cup cold pressed olive oil, or mixture of olive, safflower, sunflower
or macadamia nut
1/3 cup lemon juice
½ teaspoon whole grain mustard or mustard powder

**Combine ingredients in a screw top jar and shake well. Makes 1
cup.**
Will keep in refrigerator for about 3 days.

- Crushed clove of garlic, herbs such as thyme, basil, dill, marjoram
  /oregano
- Curried - add 2 teaspoons homemade curry powder and 2 green
  shallots finely chopped.

Italian Dressing

2/3cup cold pressed olive oil
1/3 cup lemon juice
2 crushed cloves garlic
1 small onion minced
1 tablespoon red pimiento/red pepper finely chopped

Combine ingredients in screw top jar and shake well.

Avocado Dressing

1 avocado mashed
¼ cup lemon or lime juice
½ teaspoon Dijon mustard or Homemade Seed Mustard (see Miscellaneous)
Extra juice if required

Combine all ingredients in a glass or china bowl, and stir with non-metallic spoon or spatula till smooth. The dressing will take the flavour of metal if a metal spoon is used. Set aside till required.

Orange Dressing

1/3cup cold pressed olive oil
2 teaspoons grated orange rind
¼ cup orange juice
1 organic free range egg yolk
1 tablespoon lemon juice

Blend all of the above ingredients except the oil. While blender is going, slowly trickle in the oil till the dressing thickens.

Citrus Dressing

½ cup orange juice
1 tablespoon lime or lemon juice
¼ cup cold pressed olive or macadamia oil
Dash Herbamare herbal salt
Grind of pepper (optional)
A couple of good pinches sweet paprika

**Combine ingredients in a jar and shake. Set aside till required.
Serves about 4.**

- Great served over seafood salads such as cold fish, scallops and
  prawns.

Orange Herb Dressing

½ cup cold pressed olive oil, or ½ olive and ½ macadamia oil
¼ cup orange juice
1 tablespoon lemon juice
2 tablespoons fresh thyme or 1 teaspoon dried thyme

Whisk all together and set aside till required.

Orange Dressing With a Temper

¼ cup orange juice
2 teaspoons grated rind
1/3cup cold pressed olive oil
2 tablespoons chopped parsley
1 crushed clove garlic
1 small red chilli finely chopped

Blend together all the ingredients, but the oil. With the blender still running, slowly trickle in the oil and beat till the dressing thickens.

•   In place of parsley, try coriander or another herb.

Caesar Salad Dressing

½ cup cold pressed olive oil
6 drained anchovy fillets
1 crushed clove of garlic
2 tablespoons of lemon juice
1 organic free range egg

Mash anchovies and blend all ingredients together until smooth. Set aside till required.

Thousand Island Dressing

1 cup mayonnaise (see basic mayonnaise recipe)
2 tablespoons peeled and pureed tomatoes
2 tablespoons finely chopped olives
1 tablespoon red capsicum/pepper minced
1 tablespoon pimento minced
1 tablespoon minced onion

Blend all ingredients and chill till required.

• Especially good over prawn cocktail and other seafood.

Tangy Thai Dressing

¼ cup cold pressed safflower, sunflower, macadamia or good quality sesame oil
1½ tablespoons lemon juice
1 tablespoon honey, organic maple syrup or Date Sweetener (see Miscellaneous)
1 tablespoon grated orange rind
Small piece fresh ginger crushed in garlic press (optional)
¼ teaspoon fresh ground coriander
½ teaspoon fresh ground cumin
Dash of Herbamare herbal salt
Grind of pepper

Gently heat the coriander, cumin and ginger for a minute or two to release their fragrances. Combine all ingredients in a jar, and shake vigorously. Set aside until required so that the flavour can develop. The dressing will keep two or three days, the longer kept the more developed the flavour. Serves about 4.

Coconut Dressing

1 tablespoon lemon or lime juice
1 tablespoon honey or Date Sweetener (see Miscellaneous)
½ cup coconut cream or nut cream eg macadamia, almond, cashew
nut cream
Dash of Herbamare herbal salt
Grind of pepper (optional)

**Blend the lemon/lime juice and honey, and add herbal salt and
pepper. Gradually blend in coconut cream or nut cream. Serves
about 4.**

- When coconut cream or nut creams are used in recipes, it's not
  always necessary to add sweeteners. Coconut cream and nut
  creams have a natural sweetness of their own depending on the
  nut.

Lime and Coconut Dressing

1 cup coconut cream
1 lime juiced
1 small red chilli finely chopped or sprinkle of chilli powder
2 cloves garlic crushed
1 teaspoon coriander seeds
1 teaspoon cumin seeds

**Grind together coriander and cumin seeds in a spice grinder.
Combine spices, chilli, garlic and lime juice in a small saucepan
and cook gently for a minute to allow the spices to release their
fragrance. Stir in coconut cream and heat till near to boiling,
then set aside until ready to serve. This has an excellent flavour if
left a few hours for the flavours to develop.**

- Great over coleslaw, salads of sliced carrots, grated fresh coconut,
  snow peas/mange tout, cauliflower and broccoli florets, sliced
  radishes etc.
- Use as dressing over fish such as trout, Atlantic salmon, barbecued
  Australian salmon cutlets, bream, flathead.

Pineapple Dressing

¼ cup fresh chunks of pineapple
Cold pressed olive oil or macadamia nut oil
½ lemon or lime juiced

Blend all ingredients using just enough oil to make a thick dressing.

Creamy Citrus Dressing

Juice of 2 oranges or mixture orange, lime and mandarin
½ cup coconut cream or nut creams eg macadamia, almond or cashew nut cream
1 tablespoon fresh chopped mint

Blend all ingredients to a smooth consistency and chill till ready to serve.

Simple Lemon Mustard Dressing

4 tablespoons cold pressed olive oil
2 tablespoons fresh lemon juice
½ - 1 teaspoon Home Made Mustard or Dijon mustard

Combine ingredients in a screw top jar and shake. Set aside till required. Will keep atleast three days in the refrigerator.

Oriental Dressing

½ lime, skin on, finely chopped
1/3cup fresh lime juice
¼ cup honey, organic maple syrup or ¼ cup fresh pineapple juice
could be used
2 anchovies
2 tablespoons tamarind pulp soaked in warm water for 10 minutes
and drained
¼ teaspoon chilli powder
2 tablespoons fresh coriander finely chopped
2 tablespoons fresh mint finely chopped

**Blend together the lime juice, honey/syrup or pineapple juice,
anchovies, chilli powder and tamarind pulp. Mix in chopped
lime, coriander and mint leaves. Set aside till required. Should
have a lovely sweet, sour and slightly salty taste.**

Anchovy Dressing

3 anchovy fillets finely chopped
½ cup good cold pressed olive oil
¼ cup fresh lemon juice
Grind fresh black pepper

Blend or shake together all ingredients and set aside till required.

Nut Dressing

2 teaspoons nut butter eg macadamia nut, almond butter
1 clove garlic crushed
Enough lemon or lime juice to make the right consistency

Blend ingredients and set aside till required.

- Excellent over rice salad or dishes involving egg plant.

Wholegrain Mustard Dressing

1/3cup good cold pressed extra virgin olive oil
2 tablespoons fresh lemon juice
2 teaspoons home made wholegrain mustard

Shake the ingredients together in a screw top jar. Set aside till required. Dressing will keep a couple of days in the refrigerator.

Tarragon Vinaigrette Dressing

4 tablespoons cold pressed oil eg safflower, sunflower, macadamia nut oil
3 tablespoons fresh lemon juice
1 sprig tarragon finely chopped
1 teaspoon honey or Date Sweetener (see Miscellaneous)
Dash Herbamare herbal salt or organic sea salt
Grind fresh black pepper (optional)

Combine all the ingredients in a screw top jar and shake well. Set aside till required.

Spicy Coleslaw Dressing
(Rich in spices, not hot)

1 cup coconut cream
3 tablespoons fresh lemon or lime juice
1 teaspoon honey or Date Sweetener (see Miscellaneous)
1 clove garlic crushed
1 tablespoon turmeric
1 teaspoon ground ginger
1 teaspoon cardamom
Pinch cinnamon
Pinch cayenne pepper
¼ teaspoon organic sea salt

**Gently heat the spices for a minute or so to allow the release of
their fragrances. Combine the coconut cream, lemon juice, honey
or sweetener, garlic, spices and salt and set aside till required.
Will keep 2 to 3 days in the refrigerator.**

- Delicious on coleslaw containing apple or pineapple.
- Try on hot potatoes.

Basic Mayonnaise No.1

2 organic free range egg yolks
300ml / ½pint cold pressed olive oil, or mixture of olive / macadamia
/ sunflower
  or safflower
2 tablespoons lemon or lime juice
1 teaspoon mustard powder or Home Made Mustard (see recipe in
Miscellaneous)
1 teaspoon organic honey or Date Sweetener (see Miscellaneous)

**Place all of the above ingredients except oil into a blender and
process for about a minute. Slowly drizzle in oil in a thin stream
as it processes. You will hear and notice as the mayonnaise starts
to thicken. Makes approximately 1 cupful.**

*This mayonnaise will keep in an airtight container in the refrigerator
for a few days.

Basic Mayonnaise No.2

2 organic free range egg yolks or 1 whole egg
2 teaspoons lemon or lime juice
1 teaspoon homemade mustard or Dijon mustard (optional)
1 teaspoon organic honey or Date Mixture (see Miscellaneous)
Dash of Herbamare herbal salt or organic sea salt
Cold pressed olive oil, macadamia, sunflower or safflower oil

**Blend the egg yolks, juice, mustard, honey and salt. With blender
still going, very slowly dribble in the oil until mayonnaise
thickens. The sound of the mixture blending will change. Once
the right consistency has been reached, correct the flavouring by
adding more lemon or lime juice. This will keep 3 to 4 days in the
refrigerator.**

Variations on Mayonnaise

- Add 1 clove of crushed garlic.
- Add ½ teaspoon curry powder
- Herb Mayonnaise - add chopped chives, thyme, rosemary, mint, coriander, tarragon, basil, parsley. Any of the above or a mixture.
- Chili Mayonnaise - add a ¼ teaspoon of chilli powder, chopped chillies, or a dash of Tabasco sauce.
- Add seeds e.g. dill, caraway, fennel, ground fenugreek, which gives a curry flavour without the heat, celery seeds, cumin.
- Add minced onion and / or capsicum/pepper.
- Add 1 crushed clove of garlic, 2 teaspoons fresh grated ginger and 4 tablespoons chopped coriander.

Tartare Sauce

2/3cup home made mayonnaise
3 teaspoons capers, rinsed to remove as much white vinegar as possible
2 cocktail gherkins, rinsed (try to purchase gherkins with no food coloring)
1 good teaspoon of chives

Chop capers, gherkins and chives finely and blend with mayonnaise. Refrigerate and allow the flavours to mingle.

Salmon Dressing

1 x 220gm / 7oz tin/can red salmon, drained
Tartare sauce (see recipe)
1 tablespoon chopped mint

Blend in food processor until smooth. Refrigerate till required.

- If fresh preferred, cook a salmon cutlet and use in place of tinned/canned salmon.

Dill Mayonnaise

2 organic free range egg yolks
½ cup cold pressed olive oil, or mixture of cold pressed oils
1 teaspoon lemon juice
2 tablespoons fresh dill finely chopped
Dash of Herbamare herbal seasoning salt

Place egg yolks, lemon juice and herbal salt in a blender and process until pale and thick. Add oil in a slow steady stream till mayonnaise thickens. Blend in dill. For extra tang add more lemon juice. This mayonnaise is suitable to pour over trout or salmon cutlets, or on hot potatoes.

Blood Orange Mayonnaise

2 organic free range egg yolks
2 teaspoons fresh lemon juice
1 teaspoon home made mustard or Dijon mustard
½ cup good quality cold pressed olive oil
Juice of approximately ½ a blood orange

Blend together egg yolks, lemon juice and mustard. With blender going, slowly dribble in the olive oil till the mayonnaise thickens. Quickly blend in enough blood orange juice to reach the desired taste without making mayonnaise too thin. Excellent served over citrus salads and sea foods.

Avocado Mayonnaise

1 large avocado
1 tablespoon capers finely chopped or mashed (first rinse to remove white vinegar)
1 anchovy finely chopped
1 clove garlic crushed
1 tablespoon chives finely chopped
1 lime or lemon juiced

Mash the avocado and mix in the capers, anchovy, garlic and chives. Stir in the lime or lemon juice and set aside till ready to serve.

- Dollop spoonsful on top of your favourite leafy salad. It adds a great flavour when used as a dressing for coleslaw.
- Use over seafood.

Cocktail Sauce

½ cup homemade mayonnaise
2 teaspoons lemon juice
1 teaspoon tomato paste
1 teaspoon Worcestershire Sauce
½ teaspoon tarragon
4 drops of Tabasco Sauce
½ teaspoon paprika

Blend all the ingredients and set aside till required. This sauce is especially for seafood cocktails.

Tomato Herb Sauce

4 large or 5 medium tomatoes peeled
1 small onion chopped
1 clove garlic crushed
1 tablespoon parsley chopped
1 teaspoon fresh basil chopped
½ teaspoon sweet paprika
¼ cup organic non-alcoholic and preservative-free red wine or lemon/
lime juice

**Blend all ingredients and set aside till required. Serves about 4
- 6.**

- A good sauce to use on pizza bases.
- Drizzle over cabbage rolls
- Use over tacos, tortillas or pasta

Tomato and Garlic Sauce

1 large tomato peeled and roughly chopped
3 cloves garlic crushed
50gms / 2oz almond meal
5 tablespoons good cold pressed olive oil
1 tablespoon organic apple cider vinegar or lemon juice (my
preference is lemon juice)
1 teaspoon paprika
Dash Herbamare herbal salt or organic sea salt
Grind fresh pepper (optional)

**In a blender or food processor, puree the garlic, tomato and
almond meal. Add the paprika, seasonings to taste and vinegar
or lemon juice, and blend further. With processor still running,
slowly drizzle in the olive oil. Set aside till required.**

- A good sauce for fish and as the tomato base to give lots of flavour
  to pizza. Try on salads also.
- Drizzle over cabbage rolls.
- Use on tacos or tortillas.

Hollandaise Sauce

4 organic free range egg yolks
125gms / 4oz butter or ghee
1½ tablespoons lemon juice
Organic sea salt
Grind fresh pepper

Divide butter/ghee into three roughly equal quantities and place 1/3 in the top of a double boiler with the egg yolks. Gently cook over hot water (not boiling) stirring all the time until the butter/ghee melts. Stir in second chunk of butter/ghee. This time you'll notice sauce start to thicken. Add final third of butter/ghee and stir quickly till melted. Remove saucepan from the hot water and keep beating a couple of minutes, finally adding the lemon juice, a teaspoonful at a time. Season with organic sea salt and fresh pepper.

- This sauce may seem a little time consuming but the taste is well worth the effort. And if you're wondering why we need to add the ingredients to the egg yolks slowly, we have to be careful so that our mixture won't curdle.
- Hollandaise sauce is a great addition to sea foods, egg dishes, potato salads, normal salads of vegetables, coleslaw, or hot potatoes. Just use your imagination. It's a sauce that will turn a simple dish into a gourmet's delight, especially to impress friends when you secretly serve food from your diet. Haven't you had the comment, "to eat salads and raw food all the time would be boring"? We have that said to us frequently.

Carrot Puree

500gms / 1lb fresh carrots chopped
3 tablespoons orange juice
1 tablespoon finely chopped tarragon
1 organic free range egg white
Dash organic sea salt

In a food processor puree the carrot, add the orange juice and tarragon. In a separate bowl, beat the egg white and salt until white peaks are formed, then mix into the carrot puree. Serve with fish, eggs, even dollop on top of your favourite salad.

- In place of the tarragon, add lemon verbena or lemon balm leaves finely chopped.
- As carrot is sweet, lime juice in place of orange juice will add a 'sweet and sour' taste, and grated rind of the lime will give an exotic flavour.
- In place of tarragon add a grating of a nutmeg.

SWEETS

The piece d resistance to round
off the meal and add great
nutritional value

A mixture of any kind of chopped fruit will make a delicious grand
finale' to a good meal. Add grated fresh coconut for extra nutrition
and a wonderful flavour, add a sprig of mint for refreshing taste
and as an aid to digestion. It's best to eat fruits in season and try to
buy organic wherever possible. For a change, make fruit salad from
dried fruits (look for natural sulphur-free dried fruits and beware
of the dried fruits that have been treated with sugar before hand).
Fruit salads and sorbets can be made from any combinations of
fresh fruits that may appeal to you. Sprinkle chopped nuts, seeds or
fresh coconut curls for garnish and added nutrition. For an exotic
flavour add powdered ginger, fresh ground allspice, cinnamon or a
touch of powdered cloves.

Tropical Fruit Dessert

½ pineapple peeled and chopped into chunks
1 - 2 mangoes or small paw paw/papaya, peeled and chopped into
chunks
2 peaches peeled and chopped
2 tablespoon grated or shredded fresh coconut

Blend all ingredients but the coconut, in a food processor until
smooth. Serve in glass dishes and sprinkle with fresh coconut.
For a hot summer's day, first chill the fruit in the refrigerator so
it's cool when served.

• For a creamier, smooth dessert add a ripe banana. Makes a rich
   dessert.

Tropical Fruit Salad

½ pineapple finely chopped
1 - 2 mangoes finely chopped
¼-½ paw paw/papaya finely chopped
Strawberries or raspberries
Fresh coconut water, drained from coconut and strained (optional)
Fresh coconut grated or shredded

Gently combine all fruits in a bowl with fresh coconut water, and leave for about an hour for flavours to develop. Serve in glass dishes decorated with grated fresh coconut.

- Dollop with coconut cream etc - see suggestions at the end of Sweets Section.

Fresh Fruit Salad

2 bananas sliced
1 apple either red or green diced
1 pear diced
1 orange or 2 mandarins segmented and halved
2 kiwifruit peeled, quartered lengthways and sliced
Squeeze of lime or lemon juice
Sprig of mint

Combine all but the mint in a bowl, and toss gently with lime or lemon juice to stop fruit oxidizing. Garnish with sprig of mint, cover and set aside till required.

- Any combination of fresh fruit can be used in fruit salad. It's only limited by your imagination.
- Chop some mint or lemon balm and gently mix through.

A Gourmet's Fruit Salad

½ paw paw/papaya peeled and diced
¼ fresh pineapple cubed
3 kiwifruit peeled, quartered and sliced
2 bananas sliced
250gms / 8oz strawberries hulled and sliced
2 cups grapes
3 - 4 passion fruit
Sprig of mint chopped
1 lime or lemon juiced
Nasturtium flowers for garnish

Combine all of the above ingredients in a large decorative serving bowl and toss gently. Garnish with nasturtium flowers. Cover and set aside till ready to serve. Serves about 6 - 8.

Apple and Berry Sorbet

4 dessert apples peeled, cored and roughly chopped
1 punnet / 8oz of strawberries, raspberries or blackberries hulled

Blend fruit in a food processor and freeze in trays. Every half hour or so take mixture from the freezer and stir to make sorbet more light. Serve in glass dishes garnished with small sprigs of mint.

Pear and Grapefruit Sorbet

4 ripe pears peeled, cored and roughly chopped
2 grapefruit juiced

Blend fruit and grapefruit juice in a food processor and freeze in freezer trays. Every half hour or so take from freezer and give a stir to make sorbet fluff up lightly. Serve in glass dishes and garnish with small sprigs of mint.

Aromatic Apples

4 - 5 apples cored and diced
100gms / 4oz fresh dates stoned and chopped, or dried figs chopped
Juice of a lemon or lime
1 tablespoons honey or Date Sweetener (see Miscellaneous)
2 tablespoons rose water
Fresh rose petals

**Toss apple in lemon juice to prevent discolouring. Add dates. Stir
in honey or sweetener and rose water, and set aside for atleast 30
minutes to allow flavours to blend. Garnish with fresh rose petals.
Serves about 4.**

- Replace lemon or lime juice with orange juice, and replace rose
  water with orange flower water for variation.

Tropical Fruit Platter

Mangoes, paw paw/papaya, lychees, bananas, kiwifruit, custard apple
peeled and sliced
Lime or lemon juice
Powdered ginger or fresh ground allspice
Small sprigs of mint

**Place fruit slices decoratively onto a platter, sprinkle with lime or
lemon juice and a little ginger or allspice. Garnish with sprig of
mint.**

Raw Apple Pie

Crust
2 cups almonds ground finely, or a mix of almonds, hazel, macadamias nuts
¾ cup sultanas
1 tablespoon of honey or Date Sweetener (see Miscellaneous)
1 tablespoon coconut flour (delicious, but optional)
Little water to bind if necessary
Cinnamon or allspice (optional)

Combine above ingredients in a food processor until blended, and press into pie dish. Refrigerate while preparing the filling.

- Can be pressed into individual sweets dishes
- In place of butter/ghee try macadamia nut oil or apricot kernel oil

Filling
5 apples grated
2/3 cup currants
Squeeze of lemon, lime or orange juice
Zest of 1 lemon
3 fresh passion fruit (optional)
Sprig of mint or lemon balm

Combine the above ingredients and spoon into the piecrust. Drizzle with passion fruit and garnish with sprig of mint. Refrigerate till ready to serve.

Other Fillings
- Leave out the currants above, and add to grated apple a sprinkle of either fresh ground allspice, powdered cloves or cinnamon.
- 5 - 6 peaches finely chopped, passion fruit, squeeze of lemon, cinnamon or allspice and sprig of mint
- Apple and blackberries or raspberries
- Strawberries sliced and placed in individual bases, sprigs of mint
- 3 - 4 mangoes cubed, garnished with mint and fresh coconut

curls, drizzled with passionfruit
- Substitute apples with pears
- Pineapple finely chopped, grated fresh coconut, drizzled with passion fruit, garnished with mint
- Bananas and dates with a squeeze of lime or orange juice, decorate with fresh coconut curls

Raw Carob and Minted Apple Pie

Base
2 cups almond meal or other ground nuts eg macadamias, hazelnuts
2 tablespoons carob powder
1 tablespoon coconut flour (delicious, but optional)
1 tablespoon organic honey, maple syrup or Date Sweetener (see Miscellaneous)
A little water to bind if too dry
Dash natural vanilla essence (optional)

Filling
5 - 6 apples grated
Juice ½ fresh orange, use lime or lemon if not available
2 tablespoons chopped fresh mint
3 passion fruit to drizzle
Mint sprig for garnish

Combine the *Base* ingredients in a whiz or blender, or with a spoon in a bowl. Press out into a pie plate and refrigerate until filling is prepared. Mix together the grated apple and chopped mint, then squeeze over the orange juice to prevent the browning (oxidizing) of the apple. Fill prepared piecrust with the apple mixture and drizzle over the passion fruit. If the seeds are not liked just strain through a coarse strainer. Decorate with the sprig of mint and refrigerate again till required at table.

Other fillings
- A variation to this very refreshing finish to a good meal, in place of mint add grated rind of a lime or lemon. Garnish with a sprig of lemon balm.
- Replace mint with finely chopped lemon balm.
- For a taste of the east, replace mint with finely chopped fresh kaffir lime leaves and a sprinkle of mixed spice.
- In place of orange juice sprinkle over a tablespoon of rose water or orange blossom water.
- Try with 2 - 3 tablespoons sultanas

* With these pie bases you can add any filling you like, just think about your favourite fruit combinations and it will probably work.

Berry Flan

Crust
2 cups hazelnuts ground finely
2 tablespoons organic honey or Date Sweetener (see Miscellaneous)
1 tablespoon lemon juice

Blend hazelnuts, honey/Date Sweetener and lemon juice and press into 20cm / 8in. flan tin and refrigerate.

Filling
250gms / 8oz strawberries
250gms / 8oz raspberries
A sprinkle of cinnamon or fresh ground allspice to taste
Sprig of mint

Reserve a few berries for decoration, then puree the remainder of the berries in the blender or food processor. Add spice to taste. Spoon into flan, decorate with reserved berries and mint sprig, and refrigerate till required.

* As with Apple Pie, any mixture of fruits will make a delicious flan. Try berries and apples, pears, bananas and dates etc, sprinkle top with chopped nuts or fresh coconut curls.
* Dollop with coconut cream or suggested toppings at the end of Sweets Section.

Exotic Fruit Salad

250gms / 8oz natural dried figs
250gms / 8oz sulphur-free dried peaches, apricots, apples or pears
250gms / 8oz sulphur-free prunes
150gms / 5oz natural raisins
100gms / 3oz raw, shelled pistachios
100gms / 3oz pine nuts
1 tablespoon rose water
1 tablespoon orange flower water
Filtered water

Place fruits and nuts in a china or glass bowl. Cover with filtered water, orange flower water and rose water, and allow to stand for minimum 24 hours so that the fruit can absorb the liquid and the flavour can develop.

- Garnish with coconut curls or a dollop of coconut cream.
- Serve for a special breakfast.

Fruit Kebabs

1 pineapple peeled and chopped into chunks
300gms / 10oz strawberries
4 bananas chopped into large pieces
4 kiwifruit peeled and quartered
½ cup orange juice
1 teaspoon grated orange rind
1 tablespoon lemon or lime juice
¼ cup organic honey or Date Sweetener (see Miscellaneous)
Sprinkle of cinnamon or fresh ground allspice

Arrange fruit pieces decoratively on skewers. Combine juices, rind, honey/Date Sweetener and spice. Marinate fruit kebabs for about an hour then barbecue on grill or under griller of your stove, basting frequently while cooking.

Citrus in Syrup

3 oranges peeled, be sure to remove all pith
5 mandarins peeled
4 tangelos peeled
½ cup organic maple syrup or honey or Date Sweetener (see Miscellaneous)
1½ cups water
A 3cm piece or fresh ginger peeled and sliced thinly
2 stems of fresh lemongrass trimmed, bruised and cut into 3cm lengths
Sprigs of mint

Cut oranges into segments and segment mandarins and tangelos. In a saucepan combine water, maple syrup, ginger and lemongrass. Stir till boiling, then lower the heat and simmer for about 5 minutes, to reduce liquid slightly, while extracting the flavour from ginger and lemongrass. Allow to cool. In a large bowl, 4 small glass bowls or glasses, spoon in the citrus pieces. Remove lemongrass from syrup then pour it over citrus. Garnish with mint sprig. Serves 4.

- For syrup without maple syrup or honey use plain filtered water and Date Sweetener as appears in Miscellaneous. Take from the hotplate allow to cool a little then add a dollop of coconut cream to taste. Coconut has its own sweetness and will give an exotic flavour.
- Chop and segment citrus as above, mix through a handful of chopped mint and allow to sit a while before serving, to allow the flavours to mingle.
- Serve with a dollop of coconut cream or nut cream on top of each bowl or glass (see nut cream recipe in Miscellaneous). Also see topping suggestions at the end of Sweets Section.
- Try using this syrup on other fruits.

Berry Delight

1 punnet / 8oz strawberries hulled and quartered
1 punnet / 8oz raspberries
1 punnet / 8oz blueberries
1 cup cherries
½ cup coconut cream
2 tablespoons organic maple syrup (optional - coconut cream may be sweet enough)
Small lemon balm or mint sprigs

Combine all the berries and evenly spoon into attractive glasses or individual glass bowls. Mix together the coconut cream and maple syrup. To serve, dollop the cream mixture onto the berries, and garnish with sprigs of lemon balm or mint, or serve topped with Vanilla Egg Custard. See toward end of Sweet Section. Serves 6.

Orange Avocado Delight

2 avocadoes mashed
1 orange juiced
Grated rind of orange
1 tablespoon honey, organic maple syrup or Date Sweetener see Miscellaneous)
4 tablespoons chopped organic dried figs or dates
150mls / ¼ pint coconut cream, almond cream or macadamia cream
2 organic free range egg whites stiffly beaten
Extra strips of orange rind for garnish

In a bowl, combine the mashed avocado, orange juice and rind, honey or Date Sweetener and figs. Lightly fold in coconut or other nut creams then gently fold in the whipped egg whites. Serve in 4 individual glasses or bowls, garnish with strips of orange rind and refrigerate till required. Serves 4.

Coconut Mousse Tropicale

2 mangoes chopped
1½ cups paw paw/papaya chopped
½ cup orange juice
½ cup hot filtered water
1 tablespoon agar agar or 1 teaspoon guar gum
1 tablespoon organic maple syrup or Date Sweetener (see
Miscellaneous)
3 passion fruit
1 cup coconut cream

**Dissolve agar agar or guar gum in hot water. Puree mango
and paw paw/papaya and blend in the agar agar. Chill in the
refrigerator till set, then fold in coconut cream. Pour into glasses
or sweets bowls, drizzle with fresh passion fruit and chill till
required.**

Pineapple Avocado Gelato

1½ cups mashed avocado
¼ cup coconut cream or almond or macadamia nut cream (see end of Sweets Section)
2 tablespoons honey, organic maple syrup or Date Sweetener (see Miscellaneous)
1¼ cups fresh pineapple juice
1 lime juiced
2 organic free range egg whites stiffly whipped
Fresh pineapple chunks
2 kiwi fruit peeled, quartered then cut into thick slices
Grated lime rind for garnish

Blend avocado, coconut cream or nut cream and honey till smooth. Fold in the pineapple and lime juices then very gently the stiff egg whites. Place in an ice cream tray and freeze. When almost frozen, take out and mix again then refreeze. A few minutes before you are about to serve it, remove gelato from freezer and allow to soften slightly. Scoop into glasses or bowls and garnish with fresh pineapple chunks and kiwi fruit slices. Sprinkle on a little grated lime rind for a tangy taste. Serves 6.

- This is a health conscious person's ice cream. Wonderful served on a hot day, even for children.
- Honey and maple syrup should not really be necessary, pineapple juice should be sufficiently sweet. The honey or Date Sweetener is there for those who have a 'sweet tooth'.

Sensational Stuffed Figs

15 organic dried figs
100gms / 3oz blanched almonds
50gms / 1½oz almond meal
1/3 cup mixed citrus peel
Fresh squeezed orange juice
1 teaspoon organic honey or Date Sweetener (see Miscellaneous)

Remove the hard stems from the figs and cut a cross on top of each to allow it to open out like the petals of a flower. In a blender, process the blanched almonds and citrus peel till they are fine. By hand, mix in almond meal, honey or Date Sweetener and just enough orange juice to form a stiff dough-like consistency. Take about 2 teaspoons of mixture in your hands and shape into a small ball. Place inside the fig and press 'petals' back around. Serve as sweets with Dandelion Cardamom Coffee or Spiced Rooibos Tea.

• Replace the citrus peel with fresh grated apple and a sprinkle of cinnamon or fresh ground allspice, fresh ground cardamom to taste, or a pinch of powdered cloves. Add a dash of rose or orange flower water for a special, delicate taste.

Stuffed Apples

4 cooking apples eg Granny Smith apples
4 teaspoons organic honey, organic maple syrup or Date Sweetener
(see Miscellaneous)
1 tablespoon each of sultanas, currants and raisins
½ teaspoon grated lemon rind
½ teaspoon grated orange rind
1 teaspoon lemon juice
½ teaspoon cinnamon, fresh ground allspice or powdered cloves
Dash nutmeg

**Mix together the fruits, lemon and orange rind and cinnamon.
Core the apples and just cut skin around the middle. Fill the
apples with the fruit mixture. Drizzle a little honey, maple syrup
or Date Sweetener on top, and place in a greased oven dish to
which the lemon juice and a small amount of water has been
added (to prevent burning). Cook for about 15 to 20 minutes or
until the apples feel soft when a skewer is inserted. Serve warm as
a 'comfort' food. Serves 4.**

- Honey, maple syrup or Date Sweetener is not really necessary.
  The fruit and cinnamon have their own sweetness, but it's there
  for those who like 'sweet'.
- For a little indulgence or *that* dinner party, try **Stuffed Apples
  with Brandy Sauce.** Add 2 tablespoons organic honey, organic
  maple syrup or Date Sweetener and 1 - 2 tablespoons brandy to
  the water, in the ovenproof dish to form a syrup. Baste apples
  with the syrup once or twice while they cook.
- Drizzle over a sauce or topping, recipes toward the end of Sweet
  Section.

Baked Apples

4 Granny Smith apples
Sultanas
Organic honey or Date Sweetener (see Miscellaneous)
Dobs of butter/ghee
Nuts finely chopped and cinnamon

Make a cut around the middle of apples. Remove cores without making a hole in the bottom. Fill with sultanas, drizzle in the honey or Date Sweetener and top with nuts and dollop of butter/ghee. Sprinkle with cinnamon. Place in a greased pan or small heatproof serving bowls with water just to cover the bottom and bake in a moderate oven for 20 to 30 minutes. Serves 4.

- Dollop with coconut cream or Vanilla Egg Custard, see other toppings/sauces toward the end of Sweet Section.

Fig and Orange Tart

Crust
250gms / 8oz rice biscuits crushed
125gms / 4oz butter/ghee melted (try macadamia nut oil for those strict on dairy)
1 teaspoon cinnamon or, fresh ground allspice (optional)

Combine the above ingredients and press into 23cm flan tin with removable base. Bake in a moderate oven for about 10 minutes.

Filling
250gms / 8oz dried figs chopped
1 cup orange juice concentrate
1 teaspoon grated orange rind
90gms / 3oz butter/ghee
2 organic free range eggs

In a saucepan, place figs and orange juice and bring to boil. Simmer for about 10 minutes then add butter/ghee. Allow to cool. Stir in lightly beaten eggs and pour into biscuit crust. Bake in moderate oven for 20 minutes. Remove and set aside till required. Drizzle with Vanilla Egg Custard or a complementary sauce. See toward the end of Sweet Section.

My Mum's Banana Pancakes

1 - 2 mashed ripe bananas
1 organic free range egg lightly beaten
2 - 3 tablespoons organic fruit juice or filtered water
½ teaspoon natural vanilla essence
A dash of organic sea salt
Mixture brown rice flour, corn flour, arrowroot, potato flour, tapioca flour

Whisk together the mashed banana, egg, juice, salt and vanilla then stir in enough flour to make a medium batter. Have ready a moderately hot, oiled fry pan and drop in tablespoons of batter. When the pancake starts to gently bubble, turn with a spatula and brown the underside. Serve with a spread of butter/ghee and/ or drizzle over organic maple syrup, honey, fruit purees or raw jams (see Miscellaneous). (Honey and maple syrup are not for *Candida* people).

- For a large quantity use 2 eggs and more juice or water.
- Omit bananas and have plain or add grated apple with 1 teaspoon of cinnamon or fresh ground allspice to the mixture, or sprinkle spices on top.
- Make larger pancakes and layer with sliced fresh fruit such pears, peaches, mangoes, strawberries and top with a Vanilla Egg Custard or coconut cream dressing.
- Drizzle with a Berry Couli, see recipe toward back of Sweet Section.

Marinated Peaches or Nectarines
with Vanilla Egg Custard

500gms / 8oz peaches or nectarines sliced
2 tablespoons organic honey, organic maple syrup or Date Sweetener
(see Miscellaneous)
½ lemon juiced
1 quantity Vanilla Egg Custard (see below)
Small sprigs of lemon balm

**Combine the honey, syrup or Date Sweetener and lemon juice.
In a large bowl, gently toss the fruit with the marinade and
refrigerate for atleast an hour. Serve in sweets bowls or glasses,
drizzled with custard. Decorate with sprigs of lemon balm.**

- Try replacing lemon juice with lime, orange or even mandarin for
a delicate flavour.
- Add the grated rind for extra flavour. Try mandarin when in
season, it has such a delicate taste.

Vanilla Egg Custard

2 organic free range egg yolks, lightly whisked
1 cup rice milk or nut milk (see Miscellaneous)
1 tablespoon organic honey, maple syrup, or pear, apple or grape juice concentrate
½ vanilla bean or ½ teaspoon vanilla essence
Nutmeg

Put the rice/nut milk, honey or maple syrup and vanilla bean into a saucepan and heat. Pour the hot milk mixture in a steady stream onto the beaten egg yolks, beating all the while. Return the mixture to the pan and stir constantly over a medium heat, till the custard is thickened and coats the back of a spoon. Remove from the stove, take out the vanilla bean or add the vanilla essence and pour into small bowls and sprinkle with nutmeg.

- Use this custard as a replacement for cream on sweets. It goes well over fruit salad and other fresh fruit dishes.
- Try coconut milk in place of rice milk or nut milk.
- Egg whites left over can be used to make biscuits.

Summer Fruit Pie

Crust
½ cup ground almonds
½ cup sunflower seeds
¼ cup nut butter eg cashew, hazelnut, macadamia nut etc
¼ cup tapioca flour or arrowroot
1 cup fresh grated coconut
1 tablespoon honey or Date Sweetener (see Miscellaneous)
4 tablespoons cold pressed macadamia nut oil, sunflower or safflower oil
1 dessertspoonful carob powder
Fresh orange juice

Filling
Fresh fruit of the season, diced or chopped
Passion fruit
Mint sprig for garnish

For the crust combine all dry ingredients and knead in the nut butter, oil and honey if used. Use just enough orange juice to make a soft dough, then press into a pie dish. Refrigerate. An hour or so before serving pile fruit into piecrust and garnish by drizzling over the passion fruit. Garnish with the mint sprig in the centre.

- Fruit combinations can be as varied as you wish. Apple grated and mixed with fresh orange, lemon or lime juice, add a dash of cinnamon or good pinch of cloves. Drizzle over passion fruit, or mix through chopped fresh mint or lemon balm.
- Use a mixture of apricots, peaches, nectarines, bananas or berries with orange juice
- Drizzle with a custard or topping see toward end of Sweets Section.

Apricot Coconut Cream

1 cup sulphur-free dried apricots
1½ cups warm filtered water or use half or all orange juice
1 cup coconut cream
1 teaspoon grated orange rind
1 teaspoon grated lemon or lime rind
Pecans roughly chopped
Mint or lemon balm as garnish

Soak apricots in warm water or orange juice till soft and plump, about an hour or two. Add orange and lemon / lime rind to the apricots and puree. Mix in the coconut cream, pour into serving glasses and chill. Just before serving top with chopped pecans and mint or lemon balm.

• Try pitted prunes soaked in fruit juice for a different flavour.

Summer Delight

8 ripe peaches halved
1 punnet / 8oz of fresh berries eg raspberries, strawberries halved
2/3 cup fresh orange juice
1 teaspoon cinnamon or half teaspoon fresh ground allspice
1 teaspoon organic honey, organic maple syrup or Date Sweetener
(see Miscellaneous)
Fresh grated coconut
Sprigs of mint or lemon balm

Combine the orange juice, honey and spice to form a marinade. Add peaches and berries. Marinate for atleast 3 to 4 hours. To serve, place peach halves into serving bowls or glasses, and fill with berries. Add raspberries last so they don't crush. Pour over marinade, sprinkle with fresh coconut and serve with a sprig of mint or lemon balm.
• Substitute nectarines or pears in place of peaches.
• Dollop coconut cream sweetened with organic honey, maple syrup or Date Sweetener.
• Drizzle with Vanilla Egg Custard or a sauce. See toward end of Sweet Section.

Spiced Apple and Prune Polenta

2 sweet apples peeled and thinly sliced
½ cup prunes pitted and chopped
2½ cups organic apple, pear, grape or orange juice
1 cup polenta or cornmeal
1 teaspoon mixed spice
¼ teaspoon powdered cloves
Grated rind of a lemon

Mix the lemon rind and spices through the polenta. Bring the juice to the boil in a large saucepan and with a wooden spoon stir in polenta and spices. Reduce heat and stir constantly while it cooks for about 10 minutes. Add the apple and prunes and continue to cook for about another 5 minutes. Oil a 20cm (8 inch) round bowl or cake tin and spread the polenta mixture in, making sure the fruit is evenly distributed and it's reasonably smooth on top. Leave to sit for about 3 hours or until firm. Turn polenta out onto a tray and pop under a grill for about 5 minutes or until the edges are browned. Turn over and repeat. Serve cut into wedges, hot or cold.

- Other dried fruits can replace prunes. I've made this with many combinations. Try dried figs and ginger, apple and currants/sultanas, raisins or dates.
- Seasonal fruits such as peaches, nectarines, pears will work can replace apples.
- Sultanas, currants, lemon juice, grated lemon zest, cinnamon and mixed spice is a great Christmas or Easter special.

Quick Sweet Souffle

4 organic free range eggs separated
1 tablespoon filtered water
2 teaspoons organic honey, organic maple syrup or Date Sweetener
Pinch organic sea salt
Topping of your choice, see suggestions below

**Beat together egg yolks, water and honey or maple syrup until
thick. In a separate bowl beat egg whites and a pinch of salt, till
soft peaks form. Gently fold into egg yolk mixture. Heat a little
oil in a frypan making sure the bottom and the sides are oiled.
Pour egg mixture evenly over the pan and cook on a medium heat
till it puffs and is golden beneath. Place under a medium hot
grill to set the top. Have filling prepared and spoon onto one half
of the souffle then fold over the other half. Serve immediately.
Serves 2.**

*For each serving allow 2 eggs per person and a little more water.

- Toppings can be any mixture of fruit chopped eg Sliced fresh
  strawberries, peaches, apricots, apple coarsely grated and flavoured
  with cinnamon, allspice or a pinch of cloves to taste. Add a
  handful of sultanas, sliced pears, mango, banana sprinkled with
  cinnamon and chopped macadamia nuts or almonds, sliced fresh
  figs are superb. For a big indulgence marinate fresh fruit in a dash
  of rum, brandy, Cointreau or Grand Marnier (special gourmet
  treat only, not for *Candida* people).
- Dollop with coconut cream to which a dash of organic honey,
  organic maple syrup or Date Sweetener has been added.
- Dried fruits such as apricots, figs, raisins, sultanas, prunes,
  plumped in orange juice, orange flower or rose water or hot water.
- Puree the above dried fruits in a blender and gently fold through
  the egg mixture before pouring into the pan to set.

Suggested Creams for Sweets

Dollop with some coconut cream or nut cream flavoured with lemon, lime, orange or even mandarin juice; try flavoured with natural vanilla essence, orange flower or rose water; add some allspice, cinnamon, powdered cloves. Sprinkle nutmeg on top.

Quick Coconut Cream for Sweets

Coconut cream
Organic honey, organic maple syrup or Date Sweetener (see Miscellaneous)

Blend together till smooth, and dollop on sweets.

Berry or Fruit Couli
(sauce)

Berries - strawberries, raspberries, blackberries, blueberries
    or
Soft fruit - peaches, nectarines, mangoes, paw paw/papaya, pears, apples
Dash of lime, lemon or orange juice if desired
Zest of lemon, lime, orange or mandarin

Puree your chosen fruit with lime, lemon or orange juice and rind. Serve over sweets or other fruits to make a delightful, colourful sweet. Serve swirled around the sweet on the plate and dusted with cinnamon, fresh ground nutmeg, pinch of cloves or fresh ground allspice, or drizzle over sweets such as Quick Sweet Souffle.

Sweet Avocado Coconut Sauce

1 avocado
1 cup coconut cream
2 teaspoons honey, organic maple syrup, 1 - 2 tablespoon organic
    grape juice or apple/pear juice concentrate or Date Sweetener
A dash of natural vanilla essence (optional)

Blend the above ingredients till smooth and thick.

- Add juice and rind of ½ lime. Great over tropical fruit salad.
- Use over sweets as a replacement for cream.

Creamy Fruit Salad Sauce

1 avocado
1 soft, ripe banana
1 orange juiced
1 teaspoon honey or use Date Sweetener (see Miscellaneous)

Blend the ingredients until smooth. Great drizzled over sweets especially a bowl of fruit salad. Serves 2.

- For a different flavour add ¼ teaspoon fresh ground allspice or cinnamon.

Sweet Wine Sauce

2/3 cup organic non alcoholic preservative-free white wine
2 organic free range egg yolks
1 vanilla bean split
½ cup filtered water

Simmer the wine and vanilla bean uncovered till liquid is reduced to almost half. Remove from the heat and take out the vanilla bean. Beat together the egg yolks and water until a thick and creamy consistency then slowly pour the eggs into the wine liquid whisking constantly till sauce thickens. Drizzle over sweets or fruits served for dessert.

- In place of vanilla bean use strips of lemon, lime, orange or mandarin rind, 2 cloves or a cinnamon stick depending on the dessert.

Nut Cream

1½ cups almonds, macadamias or raw cashews
1 - 2 cups filtered water
Natural vanilla essence (optional)
Honey or Date Sweetener (see Miscellaneous) This is optional

In a processor blend the nuts, essence, sweetener and water till very smooth and the desired creamy consistency.

- Sunflower seeds can be used as a replacement for nuts.

DRINKS AND BEVERAGES

Lots of nutrition can be gained from a drink. Fresh juices are the best and most pure forms of beverages, rich in minerals, vitamins and many trace elements. Carrot is excellent as a base for juices with other vegetables and fruits added. Following are some ideas for exciting, energising healthy drinks.

Fruit and Vegetable Juice Drinks

- Apple and celery - rich in minerals
- Carrot, apple and celery, very cooling on a hot day. It naturally replaces salts and potassium lost through perspiration.
- Apple and pineapple
- Orange and grapefruit or plain grapefruit - grapefruit is very alkaline.
- Carrot and beetroot or carrot, beetroot and spinach/silverbeet - a liver and blood tonic, excellent for healthy hormones.
- Carrot, apple and cabbage for the bowel
- Add garlic for a natural antibiotic, powerful antifungal and cleanser. A valuable food for *Candida* sufferers.
- Add fresh ginger, another powerful antifungal, good for circulation, digestion and great for preventing motion sickness and nausea, and will take away a headache.

The list goes on… For extra help try to purchase a copy of *Raw Vegetable and Fruit Juices* by Dr NW Walker D.Sc. He explains how to use fresh vegetable juices to solve our health problems.

My Favourite Lemon Tea

1 long piece of lemon grass top
1- 2 sprigs lemon balm torn into pieces
1- 2 sprigs catnip torn into pieces
4 leaves lemon verbena torn into pieces

Place all into a teapot and pour on 3 - 4 cups of boiling filtered water. Leave to steep for 5 - 10 minutes. Pour into cups and drink.

- Lemon balm is a soothing and calming herb, lemon grass and lemon verbena are for digestion, respiratory system and are also calmatives, and catnip is a good tonic for hormones.
- For women of menopausal age and for male hormones, add a small sprig of sage or a ½ teaspoon of dried sage. A tea with catnip and sage together, taken daily will keep hormones healthy and regulated. We often drink this for breakfast.
- Frequently we add a small sprig of fresh thyme to our tea because it has antiseptic and anti-fungal properties, beneficial for people with *Candida Albicans* to drink.

Ginger Tea
For good circulation

3 slices fresh ginger per cup
Boiling filtered water
Honey to taste - optional only for the 'sweet tooth'. (*Candida* people should definitely not have)

Place the required amount of ginger into a teapot or each cup. Pour on boiling filtered water. Allow to steep 5 - 10 minutes, then serve.

- Powerful antifungal, it is warming and aids in good circulation, particularly during winter. Prevents motion sickness, morning sickness and nausea. Serve at breakfast or following dinner at night.
- We have young children who visit us regularly and they drink this tea, without the honey, and love it.

Dandelion Cardamom Coffee

1½ tablespoons roasted ground dandelion root coffee
2 cardamom pods partly cracked to expose the seeds
1 litre of filtered water

Place the ingredients into a saucepan and simmer for atleast 5 minutes. Strain into cups and serve.

- For a refreshing after dinner drink add some fresh mint leaves to taste. Serve with a small plate of fresh dates, organic dried figs or prunes.
- Dandelion is an excellent blood and liver tonic.

Spiced Rooibos Tea

2 level teaspoons rooibos tea leaves
2 cups filtered water
½ vanilla bean split
Thin slithers of lemon or lime zest
Honey to taste (optional)

Combine ingredients in a saucepan and simmer for about 10 minutes. Strain into cups or heat resistant glasses. Sweeten to taste with honey if desired. Serves 2.

- If vanilla bean is hard to find (usually at health food stores or bulk food / organic stores) substitute with a half cinnamon stick, or whole allspice slightly cracked.

Tropical Smoothie

1 avocado roughly chopped
½ mango roughly chopped
¼ cup paw paw/papaya roughly chopped (with some papaya seeds as well)
1 banana chopped
1 tablespoon grated fresh coconut or coconut flour
2 cups fresh orange juice and/or water from fresh coconut
4 - 6 mint leaves with extra leaves for garnish
Nutmeg

Blend together all ingredients but the nutmeg. Pour into tall glasses and grate nutmeg on top. Garnish with a mint leaf and a fancy straw. Serves about 4.

- Highly nutritious for all, small toddlers and children love it, without the nutmeg of course.
- Have the fruit chilled in the refrigerator during hot summer weather and the smoothie will be refreshingly cool.
- This can still be made in winter even when mangoes are out of season, merely omit the mango, and add a ripe pear, or custard apple or increase the amount of the very nutritious paw paw/ papaya.

Banana and Orange Smoothie

1 ripe banana roughly chopped into chunks
1 cup fresh orange juice
1 organic free range egg
Cinnamon or nutmeg
Drizzle of natural honey or Date Sweetener (optional)

Place all ingredients in blender and process till smooth. Pour into glasses and garnish with suitable garnish.

Mango and Apple Smoothie

1 ripe mango peeled and cut from seed into chunks
1 cup fresh apple juice
1 organic free range egg
Dash of fresh ground allspice (optional)

Blend ingredients in processor till smooth. Pour into glasses and garnish with sprig of mint.

- Add nut milk or fresh coconut water and you have a rich liquid meal.

Banana Smoothie

1 banana chopped into rough chunks
1 cup fresh apple or pear juice, or organic juices
1 organic free range egg
1 tablespoon almond meal, or other nut meal
½ teaspoon vanilla
Cinnamon or fresh ground allspice (optional)

Blend all ingredients in food processor till smooth. Pour into glasses and garnish with apple and banana slices.

- Add any fruits to this smoothie - strawberries or any of the berries, with bananas, pears, kiwifruit, avocado …

Strawberry Smoothie

1 punnet / 8oz organic strawberries (these have the best flavour)
2 cups fresh apple or pear juice
1 banana roughly chopped
1 tablespoon coconut flour
Fresh water from a coconut (optional but extremely nutritious) or nut milk
Mint leaves or lemon balm leaves

In a blender, puree all ingredients till smooth. Pour into tall glasses and serve.

- Most fruits can be used - any of the berries, with bananas, pears, kiwifruit etc

Orange and Avocado Smoothie

1 avocado roughly chopped
2 oranges juiced
1 large organic free range egg
2 teaspoons organic honey, organic maple syrup or Date Sweetener (see Miscellaneous)
Dash of cinnamon or fresh grated nutmeg
Strips of orange rind gently tied in a twist for decoration

Blend together all ingredients except cinnamon or nutmeg. Pour into two tall glasses, sprinkle with cinnamon or grate over nutmeg, and serve with orange twist on the side. Serves 2.

Banana Whip

1 large ripe banana chopped
1 avocado roughly chopped
1 teaspoon organic honey, organic maple syrup or Date Sweetener
(see Miscellaneous)
3 glasses fresh apple juice or 2 of apple, 1 of fresh coconut milk or
coconut water
Sprinkle fresh ground allspice
Leaves of lemon balm or mint to serve

**Blend all together, but the allspice. Pour into tall glasses and
sprinkle with a little allspice. Garnish with lemon balm or mint
leaves. Serves 4.**

- Rather than sprinkle allspice on top add ½ teaspoon of fresh
  ground allspice with other ingredients.
- Replace fresh juice with organic bottled. This contains less
  nutritional value though.

Fresh Bloody Mary

1 cup fresh tomato juice
1 lemon juiced
Sprinkle of Herbamare herbal seasoning salt
A grind of fresh black pepper (optional)
1 teaspoon Worcestershire sauce
Crushed ice
Sprigs of mint

**Blend all ingredients together, but ice and mint. Place crushed ice
into glasses and pour over the Bloody Mary. Garnish with mint
sprigs.**

Pineappleade

1 fresh ripe pineapple peeled and pureed
1 cup filtered water
¼ cup lemon juice
Organic honey or organic maple syrup (optional - fruit should be sweet enough)
Passion fruit (optional)
Sprigs of mint

Blend pineapple, water, lemon juice and honey in food processor, stir in passion fruit and pour into glasses over crushed ice. Garnish with mint sprigs.

Grape Cocktail

750mls / 1¼ pints white unsweetened organic grape juice
500mls / ¾pint sparkling mineral water
Good dash angostura bitters (optional)
2 limes juiced
2 limes sliced
2 kiwi fruit peeled and sliced
Sprigs of mint
Green seedless organic grapes

Pour grape juice into a jug, add dash of angostura bitters, kiwi fruit, limes and mint. Leave to stand atleast an hour, then when ready to serve, add mineral water. To serve, place ice cubes in cocktail glasses, add a few grapes then pour over grape cocktail.

Pina Colada

1 cup fresh pineapple juice or unsweetened tinned/canned juice
1 cup coconut cream or milk
Crushed ice
Mint leaves

Blend pineapple juice and coconut cream, and pour over crushed ice in cocktail glasses. Decorate with a small wedge of pineapple on side of the glass and / or mint leaves.

• Add ½ cup cold tea for a refreshing summertime evening treat.

Citrus Cocktail

3 oranges juiced and rind grated
1 lemon juiced and rind grated
3 limes juiced and rind grated
2 grapefruit juiced
4 tablespoons organic honey, organic maple syrup or Date Sweetener
(see Miscellaneous)
1 750gm / 1¼ pints bottle of sparkling mineral water
Crushed ice

Combine all ingredients except mineral water and ice. Refrigerate the juice and cocktail glasses for minimum of 2 hours. When ready to serve, place crushed ice in the cocktail glasses, add mineral water to the juice and pour over cocktail. Decorate with lime or lemon slices.

Warm Winter Comfort

1 litre / 1¾pints fresh apple juice or organic, preservative-free bottled juice
4 cloves
1 stick of cinnamon

Place ingredients into a saucepan, bring to the boil and gently simmer for about 5 minutes. Pour into heat resistant glasses and serve. Serves approximately 4.

• Due to heating this really has little nutritional value other than to replace harmful beverages such as coffee and normal tea. On a cold winter's day or night it's both refreshing and warming while doing no major harm to the body.
• Add mint leaves before cooking and serve after dinner in place of coffee. Present with a small plate of fresh dates, prunes or organic dried figs.

Simple Appleade

3-4 apples chopped into wedges, Granny Smith apples are our favourite
½ lime or lemon juiced and skin grated
Pinch of powdered cloves
Mint leaves finely chopped

Juice the apples through a vegetable juicer. Combine juices, cloves and mint in a large glass jug, stir and serve at once. Enjoy the refreshing taste.

Iced Pineapple Tea

2 cups fresh pineapple juice
2 cups freshly made green tea cooled
1 tablespoon fresh lime or lemon juice
Thin slices of lime or lemon
Crushed ice made from filtered water
Mint leaves for garnish

In a tall glass jug, combine the pineapple juice, cool green tea and lemon juice. To serve place crushed ice in each glass, add a slice of lime or lemon and pour in the pineapple tea. Decorate with mint leaves.

- When making the green tea add mint leaves to give a refreshing mint flavour.

Strawberry Crush

1 punnet / 8oz fresh ripe strawberries
3 cups fresh apple juice
1 orange juiced
½ lemon juiced
Crushed ice made from filtered water

In a blender, puree strawberries then slowly add the juices. Spoon crushed ice into glasses and pour over strawberry crush. Garnish with extra strawberry halves on the rim of the glass.

- Other berries can be used in the same way.

Mint Julep Pricklewood Style

A sprig of mint per person roughly torn (to make a tea)
3 thin slices fresh ginger per person
½ lemon or lime juiced and rind grated
Honey to taste (optional)
Crushed ice from filtered water

Make a tea from the mint and ginger slices, and allow to steep for 5-10 minutes. Strain into a jug, add the lemon or lime juice and rind, and of course honey for those who must have it. Personally, we never see a need to sweeten food if it's fresh and raw, it has its own natural sweetness. Allow the mint julep to go cold and serve over crushed ice.

Orange and Pineapple Squash

4 blood oranges juiced
1 small to medium pineapple peeled, cored and roughly chopped
Crushed ice made from filtered water
Thin slices if orange to serve

In a blender or food processor, puree the pineapple chunks and add to orange juice in a large jug. Mix well. If necessary add a couple of cups of filtered water. Pour into glasses over crushed ice and serve with a slice of orange in each glass.

SPECIAL TREATS'
BISCUITS, CAKES
& NIBBLES

Savoury Rice Biscuits

3 cups brown rice flour
1½ tablespoons cold pressed sesame oil, or macadamia nut oil
¼ to ½ teaspoon Herbamare herbal salt
¾ cup water

Rub oil into flour and salt. Slowly add water to form a stiff dough. Knead well then roll into balls and flatten. Bake in moderate oven till brown, about 20 minutes.

* Brown rice flour can be replaced with cornmeal.
* These can be used with dips or wherever crackers are required.
* Glaze with a little beaten egg or water and press seeds on top for a different flavour. Try seeds such as caraway, fennel, aniseed or poppy.
* Mix seeds or even homemade curry powder in with rice flour before adding liquid.
* Try adding a lightly beaten egg and only ½ cup water.

Biscotti

3 organic eggs
1/3 cup organic honey or Date Sweetener (see Miscellaneous)
1 teaspoon vanilla essence
2 cups brown rice flour
½ cup cornflower or arrowroot
½ cup tapioca flour or potato flour
½ teaspoon aluminium-free, gluten-free baking powder
1 teaspoon bicarbonate of soda
Pinch of organic sea salt
¾ cup almonds

Sift together all dry ingredients three times to mix evenly. In a large bowl beat the eggs, honey or Date Sweetener and vanilla till light and frothy. Mix in the dry ingredients and the almonds with a table knife to form a soft dough. Divide into 3 parts and roll into log shapes in greased paper about 20cm/8in long. Place on a greased paper lined oven tray, and bake at 160°C / 325°F for about 50 minutes. Allow to cool on a cake cooler. Thinly slice the logs, and once again place the slices on a baking tray and cook for about 8 minutes each side. Cool. Makes about 50 slices.

Amaretti

150gms / 5oz almond meal
1 organic egg white
1 tablespoon organic honey, apple or pear juice concentrate or Date Sweetener
1 teaspoon natural vanilla essence
Blanched almonds extra

Whisk the egg white till frothy, add honey or substitute and vanilla, and continue to whisk just till honey is mixed through. Stir in the almond meal to form a stiff dough that can be piped onto greased paper lined baking tray with biscuit pipe. Alternatively take small teaspoonsful of mixture, roll into balls and flatten onto the tray. Press an almond into the centre of each biscuit. Leave to stand for 4 hours. Bake in a slow oven, about 150°C / 300°F for about 20 - 25 minutes until they are lightly brown. Allow to cool on the trays before storing in an airtight container.

- In place of blanched almonds, halved macadamia nuts and finely ground macadamia nut meal are a great alternative for a wonderful rich biscuit.
- Replace vanilla with lemon essence or grated lemon rind for another taste sensation.

Almond Wafers

2/3 cups brown rice flour
1/3 cup cornflour or arrowroot
¼ cup potato flour or tapioca flour
1 teaspoon guar gum or agar agar (optional)
4 organic egg whites
¼ cup organic honey, organic maple syrup, or Date Sweetener (see Miscellaneous)
1 teaspoon natural vanilla essence
150gms / 5oz almonds

Sift flours and gum three times to ensure they're evenly mixed. Beat egg whites till soft peaks form then add vanilla and honey. Fold in sifted flour alternately with the almonds, about ½ a cup at a time. Spoon into a greased loaf pan and bake in a reasonably slow oven, 140°C / 275°F for about 1 hour or until the bread shrinks away from the sides of the pan. Cool. Wrap in greaseproof paper and refrigerate over night. Using a bread knife or electric knife cut wafer-thin slices and place on a baking tray at 120°C / 225°F until completely dry and browned (approximately 20 minutes).

Aniseed Cookies

4 tablespoons organic honey or Date Sweetener (see Miscellaneous)
2 organic eggs
½ teaspoon natural vanilla essence
1 cup brown rice flour
1/3 cup cornflour or arrowroot
1/3 cup potato flour or tapioca flour
3 teaspoons aniseeds

**Sift the three flours together to ensure they're well combined.
Beat the eggs, honey and vanilla essence till light and creamy,
then stir in the sifted flours and aniseeds. Take small teaspoons
of mixture, place on a baking tray and lightly press with a fork.
Leave covered to sit for about 6 hours, then bake in an oven at
about 170°C / 375°F for 15 minutes or until golden brown.**

Viennese Cookies

½ cup cold pressed safflower, sunflower or macadamia nut oil
1 organic egg
2 tablespoons organic honey or Date Sweetener (see Miscellaneous)
½ teaspoon natural vanilla essence
75gms / 2½oz almond meal
1 cup brown rice flour
½ cup cornflour or arrowroot
½ cup potato flour or tapioca

**Sift together the three flours well. In a large bowl beat the oil,
egg, honey and essence till light and fluffy. Mix in the almond
meal and the sifted flours till well combined. Spoon mixture
into a biscuit forcer and pipe stars onto a greased baking tray.
Alternatively place small teaspoonsful onto tray and press lightly
with a fork. Bake in a moderate oven for about 15 minutes.**

Coconut Macaroons

2 organic egg whites
½ lemon juiced and rind grated
2½ tablespoons organic honey or Date Mixture (see Miscellaneous)
175gms / 6oz grated coconut

Beat egg whites till very stiff then add honey, lemon juice and lemon rind. Fold in the coconut and refrigerate for about 2 hours. Heap small teaspoonsful onto a greased oven tray and bake in a moderate oven for 10 - 15 minutes.

Nut Cake

6 organic eggs separated
500gms / 1lb nut meal (hazelnuts, almonds, macadamias, pecans, raw cashews)
2 tablespoons natural, organic honey or Date Sweetener (see Miscellaneous)
Dash of natural vanilla

Beat egg whites till stiff. In another bowl, beat together egg yolks and honey and stir in the nuts. Gently fold in egg whites. Pour into greased, lined cake tin and cook in moderate oven about 40 minutes.

- For a variation add a couple of teaspoons of mixed spice or cinnamon with the nuts
- Try adding 1 - 2 teaspoons of ground ginger with the nuts and fold through finely chopped, preserved/glaced ginger. (Rinse the syrup off with filtered water before using).
- Gently fold in grated orange, lemon or lime rind for a citrus flavor

Honey Nut Roll

1½ tablespoons cold pressed safflower, sunflower or macadamia nut oil
½ cup organic honey or Date Sweetener (see Miscellaneous)
1 organic free range egg
½ cup brown rice flour
¼ cup cornflour
¼ cup potato flour, arrowroot or tapioca flour
1 teaspoon gluten-free, aluminium-free baking powder
¼ cup rice milk, coconut milk, almond or macadamia nut milk
½ cup sultanas
½ cup walnuts chopped

Sift the dry ingredients together three times to ensure the flours and baking powder are evenly mixed. Beat together the oil, honey and egg till well combined then fold in the flours, sultanas and chopped walnuts. Spoon into a greased roll tin or *loaf tin and bake in a moderate oven for about 50 - 60 minutes. Test with a skewer and if it comes out clean then it will be cooked. Turn out on to a cake cooler and leave to cool.
*In a loaf tin the cake may cook quicker. Check after about 40 minutes.

- This is another recipe that you can try adding any dried fruits, nuts (I love macadamia nuts), spices, whatever takes your fancy.
- Add 2 tablespoons carob powder and natural vanilla essence

Carrot Cake

2 cups grated fresh carrot (2 medium carrots)
½ cup cold pressed macadamia, safflower or sunflower oil
¼ cup natural organic honey or date sweetener (see Miscellaneous)
3 organic free range eggs beaten
½ cup sultanas
½ cup mixture of sunflower seeds and walnuts chopped
1 cup brown rice flour - replace with cornmeal if rice flour is a problem
1 teaspoon aluminium-free bicarbonate of soda
2 teaspoons aluminium-free cream of tartar
2 teaspoons cinnamon
1 teaspoon natural vanilla essence

Sift the dry ingredients three times to mix evenly. Beat together the eggs, vanilla, oil and honey until thick. Add carrot, nuts and seeds then gently fold in dry ingredients. Pour into a greased, lined cake tin (I tend to use a ring tin mostly) and bake for about 35 - 45 minutes in a moderate oven.

Carrot and Carob Cake

2 cups grated fresh organic carrot (2 medium carrots)
½ cup cold pressed macadamia nut, safflower or sunflower oil
¼ cup organic honey or Date Sweetener (see Miscellaneous)
3 organic free range eggs
½ - ¾ cups sultanas
½ cup walnuts chopped
1 cup brown rice flour - use cornmeal if rice flour is a problem
3 tablespoons carob powder
2 teaspoons cream of tartar
1 teaspoon bicarbonate of soda
1 teaspoon natural vanilla essence

**Sift together the rice flour, carob powder, cream of tartar and
bicarbonate of soda three times to ensure they are well mixed.
In a large bowl, beat together the eggs, vanilla, oil and honey.
Add the carrot and chopped nuts, then sultanas. Fold in the dry
ingredients. Pour into a greased, lined ring cake tin and bake
in a moderate oven for about 35 - 45 minutes or until a skewer
inserted comes out clean.**

- This cake is just a version of my ordinary carrot cake above. I've
  found this recipe to be so versatile I've been able to add all kinds
  of ingredients to it and it turns out right.
- In place of sultanas, add chopped dates and spices such as 2
  teaspoons mixed spice or cinnamon. You might like to eat this
  hot with Vanilla Egg Custard (see Sweets section) and have Sticky
  Date Pudding! Or replace dates with dried figs.

Christmas Fruit Cake

6 dried sulphur-free apricots chopped
4 dried sulphur-free pears chopped
4 dried sulphur-free peaches chopped
¼ cup natural sultanas
4 dried figs chopped
4 dates pitted and chopped
1 banana
1 cup amaranth breakfast cereal
½ cup mixed chopped nuts - pecans, almonds, hazelnuts and seeds
- sunflower,
    pepitas/pumpkin
3 tablespoons fresh coconut grated
1 orange juiced and teaspoon of grated rind
1 lemon and teaspoon of grated rind
Spices - ¼ teaspoon each cinnamon, allspice, nutmeg

Process dried fruit, nuts, seeds and coconut in blender or food processor. Mash banana in a bowl and add grated rind, dried fruit and nuts and amaranth then stir in the juice. Spoon mixture into a lined loaf tin and refrigerate till ready to serve in pride of place, the centre of the Christmas table.

Iced Fruit Cake

1 cup organic natural sultanas
1 cup organic raisins
1 cup organic currants
1 cup dried figs
1 cup dates
1 cup sulphur-free dried apricots, peaches, nectarines, pears, pitted prunes or a mixture
2 cups fresh juice eg orange or apple
Grated fresh coconut, almond meal or macadamia nut meal
Icing (see Miscellaneous)

Soak the dried fruits in orange or apple juice till the fruit has plumped a bit, or softened, then mince in a food processor. Mix in enough grated coconut or nut meal to help bind the mixture and press into a spring form pan and leave an hour or two for the mixture to meld. When ready to ice, remove the sides of the pan and place on a serving plate. Spread icing over the cake and decorate with fresh flowers such as violets, rose or rose petals and mint leaves.

- For variation, replace currants with finely chopped glazed ginger (rinse in filtered water first) or use half a cup of currants and half a cup of chopped ginger.
- Add grated orange, lemon or lime rind for a citrus taste.

Fruit Squares

1 cup raw almonds chopped
1 cup organic sundried sultanas
1 cup natural sundried currants
1 cup natural, sulphur-free dried apricots diced
1 cup dates chopped
1 cup other naturally dried fruits diced eg. pears, apples, mango, peach, pineapple
1 teaspoon each grated lemon and orange rind
3 organic free range eggs beaten
1 tablespoon sherry, or replace with orange juice
2 tablespoons amaranth flour (can be found at health food or whole food stores)

Mix all the ingredients together well. Press into a greased lamington tin and bake 20 minutes in a very moderate oven. Cut into squares.

Fresh Fruit Tarts

1 cup pitted dates or dried figs
1 cup grated fresh coconut
2 large apples grated (my preference is Granny Smith apples)
1 large ripe banana mashed
Lemon, lime or orange juice

Mince the dates / figs and mix in the grated coconut. Flatten out on waxed lunch wrap or roll as for pastry and cut into rounds with a scone cutter or into squares. In a bowl combine the apple, banana and a good squeeze of citrus juice (to prevent them turning brown) and spread on fruit bases. Sprinkle the tops with more fresh grated coconut.

Fruit Chews

250gms / 8oz dried sulphur-free fruit - figs, apples, apricots, peaches, mango, prunes (one
    fruit only) chopped finely
2-3 cups nuts finely chopped, walnuts, macadamia, pecans, almonds
1 teaspoon grated lemon or orange rind
1 dessertspoon lemon or orange juice
1 tablespoon sugar-free jam keeping in flavour with chosen dried fruit

Mix together chopped fruit, jam, juice and rind and ¾ cup of the chopped nuts, then shape into balls and roll in the remainder of the nuts. Chill until ready to serve.

Hunza Nibbles

20 dried apricots finely chopped or other dried fruits eg prunes, figs, peaches, nectarines
1 tablespoon lemon juice or orange juice
1 - 2 teaspoons honey or Date Sweetener (see Miscellaneous)
Mixed chopped nuts or grated fresh coconut

Place apricots in a bowl, pour over just enough warm water to cover and leave to soak overnight. Next day blend together the apricots, lemon juice and honey. Work in chopped nuts or grated coconut to make into firm balls then roll in more nuts or coconut. Set aside till ready to be eaten.

- Add spices, grated rind, finely chopped mint, lemon balm or other sweet herbs.
- Add orange flower water or rose water to the water for soaking the fruit.

Date and Pecan Nibbles

2 cups dates pitted and minced
½ cup pecans crushed
Sprinkle of fresh ground allspice
Grated coconut

Mix together the dates and pecans. Take spoonsful of mixture and form into balls. Roll in grated coconut. Seeds such as poppy, or carob powder, are tasty alternatives to coconut.

Fruit Nibbles

1 cup sulphur-free dried apricots, mangoes, pears or apples etc
¼ cup fresh grated coconut
Orange juice
Crushed raw almonds

Soak fruit overnight in filtered water. Drain. Combine fruit, coconut and enough orange juice in food processor to make a firm dough. Form into balls and roll in crushed almonds.

Apple Bites

3 - 4 Granny Smith apples peeled and cored
½ cup fresh grated coconut
½ cup natural raisins, chopped if they are large
¼ cup each of sunflower seeds, pepitas/pumpkin seeds and sesame seeds
¼ teaspoon fresh ground nutmeg
¼ teaspoon powdered cloves
1 teaspoon cinnamon

Grind seeds finely. Puree apples and add spices, raisins, coconut and ground seeds. Form mixture into balls and roll in extra coconut. Chill in refrigerator.

Fruit Balls

1 cup dried fruits - sulphur-free apricots, organic prunes, apples, peaches, mangoes,
    pears, figs, chopped and processed
1½ cups nut mixture - almonds, hazelnut, pecans, cashews finely ground
¾ cups sunflower seeds finely ground
¼ cup sesame seeds ground
3 tablespoons fresh coconut grated
2 tablespoons natural organic honey
Juice of ½ orange
1 teaspoon grated orange rind
Sesame seeds or carob powder to coat

Place dried fruits, nuts and seeds into food processor, add coconut, grated orange rind, honey and some of orange juice and process. The mixture will be sticky. Take small amounts and roll in sesame seeds or carob powder to coat. Keep in refrigerator till required.

BREADS, SCONES & FRITTERS

Damper is the bread of the Australian cattle and sheep drovers. They made it fresh each day as a substitute for bread while droving cattle or sheep in the outback 'in the long paddock'. (Outback 'in the long paddock' was the term given to the grazing of livestock along the roadside to keep them alive in drought, or if they were being taken to market which could take weeks or even months). Damper can be cooked successfully in a camp oven or old saucepan in the coals of a fire for the same length of time as you would in the home oven. Once the fire has died down and there are good hot embers remaining, place the camp oven or saucepan in the coals. Add the damper, put the lid on and scoop hot coals onto the lid to give an even heat. I usually place the damper in on two or three layers of brown paper bags or a few layers of greaseproof paper to prevent any burning on the bottom. A bed of brown rice flour will achieve the same. Don't remove the lid until atleast half an hour is up.

Guar gum is used in some of the baking recipes because the gluten in wheat, rye, oats, barley, millet and a very similar protein in buckwheat is the 'glue' that holds breads and cakes together. This 'glue' is the problem for Coeliacs, people with allergies and intolerances and other digestive problems such as Irritable Bowel Syndrome. You can replace the water with rice milk or nut milks if you wish but in the bush, the drovers would mostly have used water.

So much can be done with a basic damper recipe. It's up to you and your ingenuity as a cook as to the different dampers you can invent. I've just put down a few of the exciting dampers I've cooked, that my family and friends have enjoyed.

Basic Damper or Scones

2 cups brown rice flour
½ cup cornflower or arrowroot
½ cup potato flour or tapioca flour
1 level teaspoon guar gum (optional)
3 rounded teaspoons aluminium/wheat free baking powder
½ teaspoon of organic sea salt or Herbamare herbal salt
1¼ cups filtered water or a little more if required

Sift dry ingredients into a bowl three times to evenly mix the baking powder and flours. Make a well in the centre and gently pour in the water. Using a table knife stir in the middle gradually incorporating more of the flour. Once most of the flour is mixed in and the dough is able to be handled, knead in the remainder of the flour till reasonably smooth. It will look like a hob of bread. Lightly cut an X on the top of the damper with a knife and place on a greased or floured tray. Bake on the bottom shelf of the oven at about 200°C / 400°F for ½ an hour. It will be cooked if it sounds hollow when tapped on top. Leave to cool a little before slicing.

*Any of these dampers can be cooked as scones or cooked in small terracotta plant pots that have been lined with greaseproof paper.

Additions to Basic Damper or Scone Recipe

- To form into scones, with the palm of your hand flatten your hob of damper out to about 3cm/1½ ins thick. Cut with a scone cutter or cut into squares and place on a greased or floured tray as for damper. Cook in a hot oven for about 10 -15 minutes. Try rolling into balls and cooking in small terracotta plant pots. They are a great novelty to serve guests.
- Add about a cup of sultanas or chopped dates and a tablespoon of organic honey, maple syrup or Date Sweetener (optional).
- Try a cup of chopped organic dried apricots and ½ cup chopped pecans
- One finely chopped onion, a teaspoon of mixed herbs and olives and / or organic dried tomatoes chopped and mixed through.
- To basic recipe add 1 cup of sun-dried tomatoes chopped, 1 onion finely chopped, 1 teaspoon of finely chopped chilli (optional), and 2 teaspoons chopped fresh herbs such as thyme, oregano or rosemary, 1 tablespoon tomato paste, mix with the water to be add to dry ingredients (optional - this does make it rich). The tomato, onion and herbs can be added to the flours before the liquid is added.
- Add savoury ingredients such as crushed cloves of garlic, finely chopped onion or herbs and spices, and flatten out as with Indian naan bread.

Pumpkin Damper

1 cup mashed cooked pumpkin
2 cups brown rice flour
½ cup cornflour or arrowroot
½ cup potato flour or tapioca flour
3 rounded teaspoons aluminium/wheat free baking powder
1 level teaspoon guar gum (optional)
½ teaspoon organic sea salt or Herbamare herbal salt
1 teaspoon fresh ground cardamom (optional)
1/3 cup of filtered water, a little more if pumpkin is dry

**Sift all the dry ingredients into a bowl three times to ensure
flours, guar gum, salt and baking powder are evenly distributed.
Make a well in the centre and add the mashed pumpkin and
water. With a table knife stir in the middle, slowly incorporating
the dry ingredients. When it starts to form a soft dough, knead
lightly with hands till all flour is used. Form into a hob, place on
a greased or floured tray in an oven at 200°C / 400°F for about
30-40 minutes or when tapped on top it sounds hollow. Leave to
cool a little before slicing.**

• In place of cardamom try mixed herbs, aniseed, caraway, fennel,
  poppy seeds, sunflower seeds, pepita/pumpkin seeds or glaze the
  top of damper with water and press pumpkin seeds on top.
• Add 1 cup sultanas or chopped dates to mixture.

My Favourite - Orange Damper

2 cups brown rice flour
½ cup cornflour or arrowroot
½ cup potato flour or tapioca flour
3 rounded teaspoons baking powder, aluminium/wheat free
1 level teaspoon guar gum (optional)
1 cup fresh orange juice
1 tablespoon honey or Date Sweetener (see Miscellaneous)
Grated rind of 2 oranges

Sift together dry ingredients three times, add the grated rind and stir through. In the centre of the flours make a well and pour in the orange juice, honey or Date Sweetener. With a table knife gently stir in the middle slowly incorporating the dry ingredients. If mixture is a bit dry just add a little water as you stir. When mixture reaches a stage that it can be handled, knead with the hands until all the flour is used. Form into a hob and mark an X on top with a knife or place small balls of dough into terracotta flower pots for individual dampers. Bake on the bottom of a hot oven at 200°C / 400°F for 30 minutes or till it sounds hollow when tapped on top.

- Try a mixture of orange and lime juice with grated lime rind for variation.
- With a pastry brush, moisten top of damper with a little juice or water and sprinkle with poppy seeds or mix poppy seeds through the damper - about 1/3 cup to dry ingredients.

Fruit Filled Damper

1 quantity of basic damper ready to cook

Filling
125gms / 4oz dried figs chopped
75gms / 2½ oz raisins
100gms / 3½ oz almonds finely chopped
75gms / 2½ oz walnuts finely chopped
1 fresh orange juiced
1 tablespoon grated orange rind
1 teaspoon cinnamon
¼ teaspoon ground cloves

In a bowl place the chopped figs and raisins and pour over the
orange juice. Leave fruit to soften for an hour or two. Mix in the
remaining filling ingredients. Roughly flatten out the damper
to about a 2cm/1in. thick circle. Heap the fruit and nut mixture
on one half of the circle leaving an edge around. Moisten the
edge with a little water and fold the other half of damper over to
enclose the fruit filling. Cut diagonals decoratively across the top.
Cook on the bottom shelf of a hot oven for the required half hour
or till it sounds hollow when tapped. Leave to cool a little before
slicing.

My Christmas or Easter Damper

2 cups brown rice flour
½ cup cornflour or arrowroot
½ cup potato flour or tapioca flour
3 rounded teaspoons aluminium/wheat free baking powder,
1 level teaspoon guar gum (optional)
1 teaspoon mixed spice
½ teaspoon cinnamon
½ teaspoon nutmeg
¼ teaspoon organic sea salt
¾ cup filtered water, a little more if mixture appears too dry
¼ cup brandy or sherry or replace with orange juice)
1 tablespoon honey or Date Sweetener (see Miscellaneous)
½ cup sultanas
½ cup currants
½ cup raisins
¼ cup glazed cherries quartered
1 tablespoon grated orange and lemon rind

Sift together all dry ingredients three times. Add the dried fruits and rind and stir around so that flours coat the fruit. (This is to ensure the fruit doesn't sink to the bottom of the damper). Mix the water, brandy or juice and honey or Date Sweetener till combined, and pour into a well in the centre of dry ingredients. With a table knife carefully stir in the middle, slowly incorporating the dry ingredients till the mixture is of a consistency to be handled. Gently knead the damper into a hob shape and place on a greased oven tray. Cut an X on the top and bake on the bottom shelf of the oven at 200°C / 400°F for 30 - 40 minutes or until it sounds hollow when tapped on top. Leave to cool a little before cutting. This is a real winner every time!

• Make small amounts of damper and form into mini dampers or Easter buns and cook on a baking tray or in small terracotta flower pots. They look most appealing served at the table in their pots.

- Tasty with any mix of sulphur-free dried apricots, dried apples, prunes, figs, pears..
- For a little indulgence change brandy for a flavoured liqueur. This is optional, we don't normally consume alcohol due to the effect on the liver and other organs of the body, but in this case the alcohol is evaporated leaving the flavour.

Is It Bread? Is it a Patty?

This is a very versatile recipe I adapted from a medieval recipe book I came across. I've shaped this basic recipe into a number of breads, pastries and bases, and I've found it to be non-fail!

Basic Bread Recipe
225gms / 8oz brown rice flour
1 rounded tablespoon cornflour, arrowroot or tapioca flour
1 rounded tablespoon potato flour
1 teaspoon gluten-free baking powder
Good pinch salt
*Knob of lard (pig fat - it's great) or butter or ghee
2 organic eggs
2-3 tablespoons water

Sift into a bowl, the flours, salt and baking powder to evenly combine. Rub the lard or butter/ghee into the dry ingredients until it resembles fine breadcrumbs. Lightly whisk together the water and eggs, and pour into a well in the centre of the dry ingredients. With a table knife, mix the liquid in until the dough can be handled and kneaded. Knead lightly then shape into the desired bread, patty or base.
If you have a food processor **this bread will take all of a couple of minutes to mix. Sift the flours into the food processor, add a good knob of lard or butter/ghee, and process to rub the fat into the flour. Add in the eggs and water and further process until the mixture is ready to be removed, kneaded and shaped. For bread, shape into a small hob and cook in a moderately warm frypan. Cook about 20 minutes one side, then turn over and cook a further 10 minutes the other side or it can be cooked in the oven for 30 minutes.**
*Lard is excellent to use in cooking. The only problem at all with using lard, is the fact that it won't be organic, and will contain the chemicals the pig has been exposed to on a conventional farm. My mother used lard from time to time, as she did 'dripping', the fat

from roasting beef. Both these fats make great 'short' pastries and breads.

- To basic recipe, for savoury, add mixed herbs, chopped dried tomatoes and olives or crushed cloves of garlic; seeds such as caraway, fennel, poppy or dill. For sweet, add sultanas, currants, 1 teaspoon mixed spice, ½ teaspoon cinnamon, ½ teaspoon ginger. This would be a good bread mixture to mould into Easter buns.
- I've used this recipe to make focaccia by patting it down a little on a greased oven tray and topping it with sliced tomato, onion and olives and other toppings.
- It makes a great pizza base. With toppings, cook about 20 minutes in the oven.
- Roll out thinly and cut into rounds. Fry quickly both sides in a greased frypan to make chapatti like breads.

Corn Bread

2 cups cornmeal or polenta
2½ teaspoons aluminium-free baking powder
1 organic free range egg
1¼ cups of organic rice milk or nut milk
1 tablespoon cold pressed oil
2 - 3 tablespoons of chopped fresh chives

In a bowl, combine cornmeal, baking powder and chopped chives. Beat together egg, rice/nut milk and oil and stir into dry ingredients. Pour into a greased 29 x 18cm (11"x 7") tin and cook for 25 - 30 minutes in a moderate to hot oven. Test with a skewer to check if cooked. Serve while hot.

- Corn bread can be cooked in a muffin tin, or clean small terracotta plant pots. It will make about 10 - 12 small muffins.
- Replace chives with 1 tablespoon dried mixed herbs, finely chopped Mexican tarragon, mint, parsley, crushed garlic or chilli.
- Mix in a tablespoon of grated orange, mandarin, lemon or lime rind.

Chapattis

2 cups brown rice flour
½ cup potato flour or tapioca flour
½ cup cornflour or arrowroot
1/3 cup cold pressed safflower, sunflower, olive oil or macadamia nut oil
½ teaspoon Herbamare herbal salt or organic sea salt
About 1 cup water

Sift all dry ingredients 3 times to ensure flours are well mixed then stir in the oil. Make a well in the centre and gradually stir in enough water to hold the dough together. Lightly knead the dough on a floured board till smooth, about 5 minutes. Cover dough and allow to stand 20 - 30 minutes. Divide into 5cm balls (2 inches) and pat or roll them out on a floured board to about 2 - 3 cm (1/8 inch) thick rounds. Have ready a medium hot oiled, pan or hot plate and cook turning once or twice till both sides are light brown. The chapattis can be placed on an oiled baking tray and cooked in a moderate oven. Serve warm with soups or curries etc.

• In place of water, vegetable stock can be used. (see Miscellaneous).

Plain Fritters

1 organic free range egg
3 - 4 tablespoons filtered water or organic fruit juice
Dash of organic sea salt
Brown rice flour
Potato flour or tapioca flour
Corn flour or arrowroot
1 level teaspoon wheat-free, aluminium-free baking powder to add lightness
Cold pressed oil or butter/ghee to grease the pan

Beat together egg, water and salt. Sift in the flours, pinch of salt and baking powder, and mix to make a medium, thick batter. Have ready a greased medium hot pan and pour in a tablespoonful of mixture at a time. When bubbles start to appear in the fritters, turn over to brown the other side. Place on crumbled kitchen paper to drain and cool slightly. Serve with soups, eggs, curries, vegetable stacks or make into sweets.

Fancy Fritters

The plain fritters above are so versatile you can add just about any flavour, fruit, vegetable, spice, herb or curry powder that your imagination can conjure up. Below are some of the fritters I've made over the years. You know how it is, on a cold Winter's day and you have the need for a warm comfort food with a cuppa or a hot soup! They only take minutes to make and can be ready to serve surprise guests.

- To make sweet fritters, add a tablespoon of organic honey or Date Sweetener (see Miscellaneous) and any of the sweet ingredients in the following suggestions.
- Add 1 or 2 mashed bananas. Add coconut flour.
- Add a squeeze of lemon or lime juice, about 1 teaspoon mixed spice, sultanas, raisins, chopped dates and grated lemon and orange juice and rind.
- Grated apple, sultanas or currants, sprinkle of powdered cloves or a teaspoon of cinnamon.
- Chopped dried figs and chopped glaced/preserved ginger (rinse off the syrup) with about 1 teaspoon of mixed spice.
- 1 teaspoon powdered ginger and chopped glaced/preserved ginger (rinse off syrup).
- Finely chopped peaches with a dash of fresh ground allspice.
- Chopped dried apricots.
- Add a cup full of fresh blackberries, adjust liquid quantity accordingly.
- Try grated apple and chopped prunes.
- About 1 tablespoonful of homemade curry powder with sultanas, raisins and currants. Add grated zucchini or parsnip, even carrot for a warm delight.
- For other savoury pancakes, add cooked flaked fish or seafood, chopped tomatoes, mixed herbs, garlic, onions…

MISCELLANEOUS

Pizza Base 1.

¾ cup brown rice flour
¼ cup cornflour or arrowroot
¼ cup potato flour or tapioca flour
1 teaspoon aluminium-free, gluten-free baking powder
½ teaspoon guar gum
¼ teaspoon Herbamare herbal salt or organic sea salt
1 tablespoon cold pressed olive oil
1/3 cup filtered water

**Sift the dry ingredients together 3 times to ensure they are
thoroughly mixed. Make a well in the centre of the dry
ingredients and add the water and oil. With a table knife stir in
the dry ingredients. Once it has reached a dough that you can
handle, turn out onto a floured board and knead well. Press
dough onto an oiled pizza tray (I cheat, I roll it out with a plain
drinking glass or jar) using fingers to press around edges. Top
with Tomato Herb Sauce and your favourite toppings. Bake 15
- 20 minutes on the bottom shelf of a moderately hot oven.**

- This base can be made in a food processor - place in the dry
  ingredients, add the oil and blend till mixture resembles fine
  breadcrumbs then add the water.
- Guar gum can be omitted by adding 1 beaten egg. The egg and
  the water together need to make 1/3 cup of liquid.

Pizza Base 2.

1 cup brown rice flour
½ cup cornflour or arrowroot
½ cup potato flour or tapioca flour
2 teaspoons aluminium-free, gluten-free baking powder
½ teaspoon guar gum
Dash Herbamare herbal salt or organic sea salt
1 tablespoon cold pressed olive oil
½ - ¾ cup filtered water

Sift together the dry ingredients 3 times to ensure they are well combined. In a food processor blend the oil into the dry ingredients till it resembles fine breadcrumbs. Add just enough water to form a firm dough. Roll out onto an oiled 25 - 27cm (10in) pizza tray (easy with a plain drinking glass or jar) and use finger tips to press into the edges. Top with Tomato Herb Sauce and favourite toppings. Bake on the botton shelf of a moderately hot oven for 15 - 20 minutes.

- Guar gum can be omitted by adding 1 beaten egg. The egg and water together need to make ½ cup of liquid. If dough is too dry add a little more water.

Nut Milk 1.

- from Roman Times, used as an alternative to cow's milk

125gms / 4oz fresh raw almonds or macadamia nuts
1¼ cups filtered water

Blend together the nuts and filtered water until very smooth. For feeding to your baby, strain it through fine muslin first.

Nut Milk 2.

1½ cups fresh raw almonds or macadamia nuts
4 cups filtered water
Natural vanilla essence to taste (optional)
Raw organic honey or Date Sweetener
Sprinkle of cinnamon

Blend the nuts and water till very smooth then add vanilla, honey and cinnamon. Strain through a sieve and serve.

- For a thick milk or cream add a ripe banana and puree.
- Sunflower seeds are also a healthy alternative.

Nut Butters

Nut butters are made by chopping nuts in a blender until they form a butter. Some vegetable juicers have an attachment to make nut butters also. A dash of cold pressed oil such as macadamia nut oil or almond oil sometimes is necessary to get them to a butter consistency. Excellent used in place of peanut butter for which they are a healthy, nutritious replacement.

Date Sweetener

2 - 4 dates
Orange juice, apple juice, grape juice, fresh or bottled organic, or filtered water

Soak the dates in juice or water overnight, or all day, till soft. Blend the mixture until it is very smooth, ensuring that you have enough juice to make to the consistency of honey. Use as a sweetener in recipes to replace honey or maple syrup. The dates add extra fibre and important nutrients to your food.

- Use more dates and juice to make the quantity required for your recipe. For an example, to replace ½ cup honey I put about 4 dates in a ½ cup measuring cup, topped up with fresh juice or filtered water. Soak, then blend till very smooth.

Homemade Vegetable Stock

2 potatoes, washed and chopped
2 large carrots roughly chopped
2 parsnips roughly chopped
1 large onion chopped
3 stalks celery chopped
3 sprigs parsley
2 bay leaves
Sprigs of fresh thyme, marjoram or oregano, tarragon, rosemary
½ teaspoon Herbamare herbal salt or organic sea salt
6 peppercorns
Large strip of lemon rind

Combine all ingredients in a large saucepan and cover with filtered water. Bring to the boil and gently simmer for 1 - 1½ hours. Strain stock, discard the vegetables (I give them to our animals, usually our dog) and store it in the refrigerator. It can be kept for up to 4 days. To keep longer, pour into containers in 1 or 2 cup quantities and freeze till required.

- Any vegetables can be used in the stock including broccoli, cauliflower, cabbage, sweet potato, turnip etc. Because this is cooked there is no food value in stock but it is a base that can be used in raw recipes such as soups and it sure beats buying it.

Chicken Stock

500gms / 1lb farm bred or organic chicken bones or wings
1 large onion roughly chopped
1 large carrot chopped into chunks
1 large parsnip chopped into chunks
1 stalk celery chopped into chunks
3 good sprigs parsley
1 sprig thyme
1 bay leaf
½ teaspoon Herbamare herbal salt
1 teaspoon black peppercorns

Place chicken in a large pan and cover with water. Add the other ingredients and bring to the boil. Simmer 1 - 2 hours then strain. Refrigerate until required, or freeze in measured quantities to use when called for in recipes.

- Being cooked it has no nutritive value but is a base for soups and can give flavor to other fresh, raw creations.

Homemade Curry Powder

30gms / 1oz coriander seeds ground
2 teaspoons garlic powder
1 tablespoon cumin ground
2 teaspoons ground turmeric
1 teaspoon ground ginger
1 teaspoon chilli powder (less if it needs to be moderately warm)
½ teaspoon ground allspice
½ tablespoon organic sea salt
1 tablespoon black pepper (less if it needs to be moderately warm)
½ teaspoon mustard seed ground
½ teaspoon saffron threads (optional - I never use, I'm not fond of the taste)

Grind and process all ingredients together. Store in an airtight jar.

Homemade Seed Mustard

½ cup white mustard seed
½ cup black mustard seed
½ cup ground mustard seed
½ - ¾ cup of fresh lemon juice
¼ cup honey or Date Sweetener
¼ - ½ teaspoon Herbamare herbal salt

Combine ingredients in a bowl and set aside for about 2 hours. Stir again and add more lemon juice if mustard is too dry. Store in clean jars in refrigerator. Use within a few weeks.

Lemon and Coriander Stuffing

¾ cup mixed nuts, finely chopped ie macadamia, almonds, raw cashews, pine nuts
2 tablespoons coriander finely chopped
Grated rind of lemon
½ lemon juiced
1 clove garlic crushed
2 tablespoons butter/ghee melted or cold pressed oil
1 organic egg, beaten
1 teaspoon raw organic honey or Date Sweetener
Some lemon thyme finely chopped (optional)
Good dash of Herbamare herbal salt or sea salt
Fresh ground pepper

Combine chopped nuts, lemon rind, coriander, garlic and seasonings. Mix together lemon juice, honey, melted butter/ghee or oil and beaten egg. Work into the dry ingredients and stuff into poultry cavity. Truss with string and roast.

My Favourite Stuffing

¾ cup macadamia nuts and almonds, finely chopped
2 tablespoons fresh coriander or Italian parsley, finely chopped
5 organic dried peach halves or 6 dried apricots, finely chopped
1 small onion, finely chopped
Squeeze lemon juice
Zest of lemon
1 rounded teaspoon of raw organic honey or Date Sweetener
1 organic egg lightly beaten
1 tablespoon melted butter or ghee
Dash of sea salt

In a bowl, combine the first 6 ingredients and the sea salt. Mix together the honey, beaten egg and butter/ghee and work into the dry ingredients. Fill the chicken cavity with the stuffing, and truss the bird to cook.

- Replace the lemon juice and zest with orange juice and zest. Stuff duck with the mixture for my version of Duck `a l'orange. Bake or braise by adding fresh orange juice and honey or Date Sweetener to the pan and basting the duck from time to time..
- Spoon into an ovenproof dish and cook for about 15 - 20 minutes or until it turns golden on top. Serve as an accompaniment to poultry or meat dishes.

Apricot Chutney

500gms / 1lb apricots halved and chopped
2 tart apples peeled and chopped (my favourite - Granny Smith apple)
250gms / 8oz onions thinly sliced
2 teaspoons grated fresh ginger
1/3 cup raisins
1½ cups organic apple cider vinegar
1 lemon and 1 orange juiced
2 tablespoons raw organic honey or 1/3 cup apple, pear or grape juice concentrate or
    use Date Sweetener
1 teaspoon mustard seed
Dash Herbamare herbal salt or organic sea salt
Dash cayenne pepper

In a large saucepan combine all the ingredients and bring to boil. Simmer for about 1 hour or until the fruit and vegetables are soft. Adjust seasonings to taste. While still hot pour chutney into glass jars and seal. Store away in a cool dark cupboard for about 6 - 8 weeks to allow the flavours to develop. The chutney will keep up to 6 months while sealed, but after opening should be kept in the refrigerator.

Dried Fruit Sauce

50gms / 2oz dried apple slices
50gms / 2oz dried pear slices
2 tablespoons raisins or sultanas
1 stick cinnamon
1¼ cups fresh apple juice or organic bottled juice
1¼ cups water
1 tablespoon arrowroot

**Soak the fruit overnight or all day in the juice and water. Add the
cinnamon stick and bring to the boil. Add a little water to the
arrowroot and blend to make a smooth paste, then stir into the
fruit mixture to thicken into a sauce.**

• Use with savoury rice dishes, on fritters or add to damper to make
  Indian naan bread.

Dried Fruit Spread

250gms/8oz natural sulphur-free apricots
250gms/8oz natural prunes pitted
250gms/8oz sulphur-free dried peaches, nectarines, figs, pears or
apples etc
1 cup fresh pureed pineapple

**Soak overnight in just enough filtered water to soften fruit. A
little lemon or orange juice can be added if desired. Blend all the
above ingredients in a food processor and store in refrigerator.**

Marmalade Spread

125gms / 4oz dates pitted
125gms / 4oz sundried currants
125gms / 4oz organic sundried sultanas
50gms / 2oz sundried raisins
50gms / 2oz figs
Juice of 1 orange and 1 lemon
1 teaspoon zest of both the orange and lemon

Soak dried fruits overnight or until juice is absorbed and fruit is soft. Blend in a food processor until reasonably smooth. Store in refrigerator.

Sugarless Jam

Chosen fruit - berries, peaches, apricots
¾ cups of apple, pear or grape juice concentrate to each cup of stewed fruit
Juice of a lemon

Stew fruit till soft. Measure fruit by the cup, add ¾ cups of juice concentrate and lemon juice. Cook till a little jam on a saucer sets when cold. Bottle and store in dry dark place.

Fresh Strawberry Jam

2 punnets / 8oz strawberries hulled and halved
2 tablespoons raw organic honey, maple syrup, or concentrated pear,
apple or grape juice
1 teaspoon finely chopped fresh common mint or peppermint
1 tablespoon lemon juice

**Puree all the ingredients and store in screw top jars. Use within
10 days.**

- In place of mint finely chopped lemon balm adds a wonderful
  flavour.
- Use as a sauce on other fruits for sweets or for breakfast on rice /
  corn cakes, rice or corn bread, damper, fritters or pancakes.
- Replace strawberries with other berries in season

Carrot and Apple Jam

250gms / 8oz carrots finely diced
1 tart apple eg Granny Smith apple grated or shredded
¾ cup filtered water
1 tablespoon raw organic honey, maples syrup or Date Sweetener
1 lemon juice
¼ teaspoon cinnamon

**In a saucepan, simmer the diced carrot for about 10 minutes till
soft. Puree, then add the apple, lemon juice and cinnamon, and
cook for a further couple of minutes. Allow to cool to handling
temperature then add the honey, maple syrup or Date Sweetener.
Spoon into screw top jars and store in the refrigerator. Use fresh.**

Prune Jam

250gms / 8oz organic prunes pitted and chopped
2 tablespoons walnuts finely chopped
1-2 tablespoons raw organic honey, organic maple syrup or Date
Sweetener
1-2 tablespoons lemon juice
1 tablespoon brandy
½ teaspoon cinnamon
Pinch nutmeg or grind of fresh nutmeg
Pinch ground cloves

**Puree the prunes, walnuts, 1 tablespoon honey, maple syrup
or Date Sweetener, 1 tablespoon lemon juice, liquor and spices
then adjust flavour with more lemon juice and/or honey to taste.
Spoon into screw top glass jars and store in a cool dark cupboard.
Use within a month.**

Hunza Jam

20 dried apricots or other dried fruits finely chopped
1 tablespoon lemon juice
2 teaspoons raw organic honey or Date Sweetener

**In a bowl, combine apricots and enough warm filtered water to
cover and leave to soak overnight. Next day, place in a blender,
add the lemon juice and honey or Date Sweetener, and puree.
Spread on rice cakes, damper or rice bread.**

- Use extra water or orange juice and you have a delicious sauce to
  use over sweets or other dishes. Add finely chopped mint, lemon
  balm, catnip
- Dried apricots soaked in orange juice with grated rind of orange,
  lemon or lime then pureed, makes an excellent marmalade
  flavoured jam.
- For a main meal sauce, add raisins, sultanas and some spices or
  herbs
- This recipe can be applied to any of the dried fruits. Imagine a
  plum, fig or peach sauce over your favourite dish.

Icing for Cakes

2 ripe bananas
Coconut cream or nut cream
Natural vanilla essence (optional)
1 teaspoon raw organic honey, organic maple syrup or Date
Sweetener

**Puree the bananas with enough coconut cream to make the
mixture spreadable. Add in the honey, maple syrup or Date
Sweetener if desired.**

Granny's Cough Mixture

1 tablespoon fresh lemon juice
1 tablespoon raw organic honey
1 tablespoon glycerine

**Mix together in a cup or small bowl. Take by the teaspoonful
as often as required. Glycerine soothes the throat and calms
coughing, lemon and honey break up the congestion. You can
never overdose on a natural medicine such as this. It has no toxic
chemicals, no artificial flavouring or colouring, it's cheap … and
it works!**

Suntan Lotion

**Pour ½ cup cold pressed apricot kernel oil, olive oil or macadamia
nut oil and 1 tablespoon of organic apple cider vinegar into a
dark glass jar and shake well. Apply to your skin as protection
against sunburn and the weather, always shaking before use.
Store in a dark cupboard.**

Recipes

Letters of Endorsement

3rd February 2003

My son had been sick since he was about seven weeks old. He constantly had a crackle when he breathed, rather like he was breathing through a snorkel. This would then develop to varying degrees -
- green mucous from his nose
- coughing
- vomiting
- croup
- fevers - sometimes spiking 41*c
- a febrile convulsion
- and just to make it interesting - a swollen eye and foot

I tried to treat this naturally, but once during this time he was hospitalized and given adrenaline and Redipred. He had a Panadol suppository once after the convulsion (a bit pointless really, as the convulsion had already brought his temperature down). I avoided the doctor's office as much as possible, but bent to family pressure once and was given antibiotics for bronchial pneumonia which lifted the crackle for about a week, then it returned.

A wonderful chiropractor helped me through this time (and still does) and I'm sure Jared would have been even worse without her help, but we were still baffled. Why was he getting sick? Jared was breastfed, ate pretty good food and had heaps of cuddles and love. I have always been interested in diet, we rarely ate dairy or wheat foods.

One day I saw an article in a magazine written by Beverley Southam about her book "A Primitive Diet". I had to have this book. I received it, read it, agreed with it, and continued to eat the way we had been... and Jared stayed sick.

In the midst of one of Jared's 'episodes' - listless, fever, disinterested, vomiting, I contacted Beverley who threw me a lifeline.

- What am I eating?
- What is Jared eating?
- Rye bread - sorry, out!
- Soy milk - probably not a good idea!

With her encouragement I was motivated enough, even though I was utterly exhausted, to start preparing salads for lunch and tea and fruit and nuts for breakfast.

Did Jared get better? Did he ever!

He's grown heaps, physically and emotionally. He's active, interested, basically a wonderfully healthy and strong boy.

By the way, I know it's hard to eat differently to others and I have weakened at times. At one of my daughter's school lunches, Jared grabbed a sausage roll. What harm can it do him I thought. About five seconds later he was vomiting violently - his body knew what harm it could do. Only a couple of weeks ago he was given an egg on wheat toast. For a whole week he suffered vomiting, diarrhoea and dehydration.

Jared's story is extreme but our whole family has benefited from this lifestyle. My husband and daughter eat mostly this way with a few exceptions. My husband has lost weight and uses his puffer rarely now. My daughter is more energetic and her eyes are very clear (my personal preference as a health indicator).

There are recipes here for any occasion. I recommend this book to anyone, in sickness or in health! It's the way it's meant to be.

Deb Palmer
Port Lincoln South Australia.

CRCRCRCR

17 February 2003.

Dear Bev,

Enclosed is a photo of me, baby Scarlet (8 weeks old), Don my husband, Laura (3) and Lucinda (5). My other two children Anthony (8) and Gabrielle (6) were absent in this photo. It may take a while for this letter to finally reach you because I needed to get a reprint of the photo as I can't bear to part with any of my photos!

As I mentioned to you Bev, after the initial shock of finding out I was pregnant with my fifth child I was determined to have a placid baby and be fitter and calmer during my pregnancy. I was going to do it right this time.

After reading your first book, what caught my attention were the words "colicky babies can be a result of wheat and dairy". These foods I greatly reduced during my pregnancy. I also started each day with a big glass of warm water with freshly squeezed lemon juice. I ate heaps of salads and fruit. I wasn't perfect in my diet but I was aware of foods and very conscious of binges.

People told me I looked wonderful in my pregnancy. I wasn't carrying any excess weight, felt calm and was positive about my unexpected bundle. Not bad for nearly 40 years old! The proof was 'in the pudding' when I delivered a perfect baby girl, Scarlet Genevieve, weighing 9lb 7oz *in only 2½ hours.* She arrived spot on her due date, November 3, 2002. I took no drugs, my body was not torn and I wasn't exhausted. My baby had the most beautiful skin colour, which the doctors all commented on, she breastfed well and I was up and walking to my room and showering within an hour.

Scarlet has been the most placid of my five children. She still has the odd bad day but 'sleeps like a baby'. I could have had 10 babies and labours like Scarlet's compared to 20 hour long horrific labours producing screaming, demanding babies like my previous 4 babies. I wondered if it could possibly be my life style change? I think it possibly could have!

Thanks for all your positive and caring telephone calls Bev. I'll keep up the good work.

Love

Noelene, Scarlet and family.
Crossover, Victoria.

ᘒᘒᘒᘒᘒ

20th January 2003

Dear Bev,

Thank you so much for your letter and yes please I would like your new book.

Our health has improved thank you. Dennis never had a sore throat all through winter and he usually has one all the time. He has rice milk because he doesn't like soy. I'm the opposite. My singing is better now too.

The most important thing that's happened though, is the change in my 8 year old grandson. His behaviour at school was **very** bad - bad language and violent towards other children and his teachers. He had an allergy test done and was allergic to wheat and dairy products. He has always been on soy milk since a baby but it was products with dairy in it that caused problems. After a few weeks his behaviour improved by about 80%. He is such a nice little boy now. One day before Christmas my daughter rang to say he had been suspended for 4 days from school. The first thing I said was "What has he eaten?" and it was pizza. I went crook at my daughter so did her older sister who also asked, "What has he eaten?" My daughter, his mum, is also on the diet but 'needed' some pizza. I told her to have it while the children were at school.

We were pleased to see that you have pizzas in your new book, as well as more nibbles for the children.

Thank you again
Regards

Mrs R.B.
Wagga Wagga NSW

かなかなかな

Letters From Jasmin
New York USA

29ᵗʰ March 2003

Hello,

I have a three year old son who is normal by all accounts except he has a significant speech delay. He spent two years in Speech therapy and improved a lot but has still to call me "mammy" or use sentences. His therapist and I am stumped since we can't force him to speak. I recently came across an article that said that a child's diet significantly impacts on his ability to produce speech and that Casein and Gluten may be to blame. They contain a chemical called Opiates that has a toxic reaction with the brain. Anyway, I say all that to say that I've been searching for resources to aid in changing our diets. I do not eat red meat but still consume fish. I'm completely in the dark about where to start or how to go about it. I was hoping that maybe you can assist me in that area … I really do hope you can help me. Thanks,

Jasmin

かなかなかな

30th March 2003

Hi,

I'm so happy that you wrote back to me with such great information. I'm so glad that the ball is now rolling and that I can start taking steps to help my son and eventually my whole family. My son eats a lot of cheese and drinks a lot chocolate milk, (his father was like that as a baby so my son became addicted to it in a very little time). In order to wean him I thought I could start him on soy cheese and soy milk. I really would like to just stop it altogether but I have to pick my battles carefully. What do you think? He is very picky with vegetables though he only likes carrots and green beans and everything has to be covered in tomatoes or tomato products. He loves marina sauce with sweet peppers. What about snacks, are graham crackers okay, how about potato rolls? I am always on the go so I need handy snack ideas. Do you have any suggestions? ... I am so grateful for your input...

Thanks again for your gracious help. I look forward to hearing from you soon.

Jasmin.

಼ೲೲೲೲ

4th April 2003

Hello,

Good to hear from you again. I took your advice. I took every dairy and grain product out of my pantry and took it to my church for charity, and went to the health food store to stock up on Organic produce... Anyway, I was so excited that I cooked my family including my son some steamed vegetables and freshly squeezed carrot and apple juice and grilled salmon steaks. My son only ate the fish and drank the juice, he wouldn't touch the vegetables. It's been almost a week now and we are still at a stalemate. Which is why I'm so glad you mentioned Ester C and your Naturopath. I'm in search of such a person. We visited my son's doctor and I mentioned that I was changing his diet and he nearly lost his mind. He told me all the horrible things that you mentioned, and more, he even told me that he may report me to children's services if I made 'such a drastic change'. I was a little shaken at first, but then I looked around his office on my way out and saw that it was packed with kids coughing and crying and generally cranky, and I felt that he was probably trying to scare me. I'm sticking to my guns with this diet because I'm seeing little changes in my son since I started. He is having more restful sleep and is much more pleasant that he used to be. He seems happier. I think that with continued effort he will continue to improve.

Well it was a pleasure once again, write soon.

Sincerely yours,

Jasmin.

❧❧❧❧❧

21st May 2003

Hey there, I was a little worried about you for a while, I thought something had happened to you guys, good to know that you are all okay and doing fine… Anyway, I haven't been to my doctor for a long time since that episode, and I won't be going back. My son is doing wonderfully, he has done a complete 360 and is speaking in phrases and beginning to use whole sentences more frequently. His speech therapist is amazed at his progress. We still keep her with us as we are attempting to help him along by exercising his mouth muscles by using oral cones, though I feel there must be another way to effectively do this without artificial means. Do you have any ideas of natural foods that may help our situation?

I am just amazed at Cameron's progress though, he is eating stuff he never used to and asking for seconds. You were right, take away the milk and once the Ester C kicked in, he is eating anything in front of him. He is even eating brussel sprouts!! My husband, seeing how well the rest of us are looking and feeling has changed his eating habits and has even stopped eating meat. I don't know how to thank you. The information you gave me was priceless and has saved my son from his doctor and insensitive therapists. May God bless you for this.

With love always

Jasmin and Family.

ↄ⁄ↄↄↄↄↄ

25th May 2003

Hi there,

... I had a wonderful Mother's Day also, we spent the day with my mother-in-law, cooking and eating and having lots of laughs and fun with the kids. She is so amazed at how far Cameron has come. She was skeptical at first though. She might even start changing the way she eats also.

We were so grateful for your help, I can't thank you enough. You have been a ray of hope in the sea of skeptical doctors and insensitive, jaded therapists. Before I used to spend sleepless nights worrying about the mental and physical health of my son. Now we have conversations on what he wants for dinner and what he wants to wear to school. It's like it was when we saw him for the first time when he was born, just amazement.

I'll talk to you soon.

Jasmin.

ↄ⁄ↄↄↄↄↄ

30th May 2003

How is everything Bev…

You know you spoke of your friends' baby, I remembered how panicked I was when Cameron was born, about getting him immunised. I was at the doctors every month like clockwork and he was developing fine until his MMR shot and then he just became a shell of himself. My daughter who was born a year later, because we were so preoccupied with Cameron, she missed most of her shots and she is far more advanced with speech and motor skills than he is for his age. So in essence she was spared his fate. I wish I had known someone like you when my kids were babies, we would have been spared a lot of pain and questions like "what if… and "what did I do wrong?" But that's history.

Write soon

Love Jasmin.

೧ഛಲೞಲಲ

1st June 2003

Hi there Bev,

…YOUR BOOK IS REALLY FABULOUS. I'm almost through reading it. The information about the genetic enhancement of our fruits and certain plants is really scary. I'm telling all of my friends about the info and they can't believe it. Sometimes until information like this is put in black and white we go on living in our own little bubble. My friends all had their bubble burst this week. Thanks again.

Jasmin.

Special thanks to Jasmin for allowing me to print excerpts from her letters. Her story I hope will help other parents having problems with their babies and children. It is my firm belief that diet and proper nutrition according to the Laws of Nature can overcome almost all health problems… so folk, there is hope.

12 September, 2007

Dear Bev,

Well, here we are 12 months since I staggered into your shop seeking help for a debilitating case of diverticulitis.

I had been diagnosed some 15 years ago and had put up with the pain, bloating and continuous bowel problems, sometimes to the stage where I could barely walk for the pain in my groin area. Then I had a major attack and ended up in hospital on a continual drip of massive antibiotics for 6 days, as I had a 4cm abscess in my bowel.

When I arrived home a neighbour called in. After talking to her she said, "You need to read Bev Southam's book. It will help you." I read it over that weekend, then staggered into your shop the following Monday, and said "Please can you help me?" You told me to change my diet, to get rid of all wheat, meat, dairy, bread and processed foods, and that I would have an improvement by Thursday.

Home I went with my list of what to do, feeling a little apprehensive about our talk, as I had been ill for such a long time. I stuck to your words rigidly, and by Wednesday I noticed a small improvement in myself. I thought, blow waiting for Thursday, I am going to see Bev today and tell her I am a little better. Bev still tells me she remembers the glow I had on my face that day, as I could see that the foods I was eating were 100% of my troubles.

It is a year ago now. I still buy organic, rarely 'break out' and eat something bad for me, as I know that I will pay for it for days afterwards, so I feel great. People stop me in the street and tell me how well I look, and this is all due to you, my dear friend, just taking the time to care about, talk to and help people lead a natural healthy life style.

Thank you Bev,
From

Jan
Narooma. NSW

NOTES

NOTES

NOTES

Made in the USA